BREATH OF RESILIENCE: NAVIGATING THE JOURNEY THROUGH LUNG CANCER

The Author assumes no responsibility whatsoever, under any circumstances, for any actions taken as a result of the information contained herein.

You are required to seek professional help if needed.

Preface

The shelves of bookstores are filled with many fine books on Lung Cancer. Why another one? I believe there is always a need for simple truths – no matter how often they are told

The issue of Lung Cancer has become a worrisome one to a lot of people suffering from this.

If by reading this book, a person can say" Wow, now I get it. I see something that could really help me*, then my purpose as an author has been fulfilled.

One of the greatest motivations in my own life is to see someone who has been dealing with a particular issue experience remarkable life change.

If I can help someone understand and apply the tips that he or she otherwise would have missed, then creating this book will have one of the most rewarding experience of my life.

LEO CHAMBERS

Contents

Introduction

Once upon a time, in a bustling city nestled between rolling hills and shimmering lakes, there lived a community bound together by the rhythms of daily life. It was a place where laughter echoed through cobblestone streets, where families gathered around dinner tables adorned with homemade delicacies, and where the warmth of human connection filled the air like a comforting embrace.

In this vibrant tapestry of humanity, there were stories woven into the fabric of every life—tales of triumph and tragedy, of love and loss, and of resilience in the face of adversity. But amidst the laughter and camaraderie, there lurked a shadow—a silent menace that cast a pall over the lives of those it touched.

This shadow bore a name that struck fear into the hearts of many—a name whispered in hushed tones, spoken with trembling lips, and dreaded like a specter in the night. It was a name that carried with it the weight of uncertainty, the anguish of diagnosis, and the relentless march of time—a name known to all as lung cancer.

Our story begins not with the shadow itself, but with the people whose lives were intertwined with its presence. Among them was Maria, a vibrant woman with a smile that could light up the darkest of rooms. Maria had always been the life of the party, the heart and soul of her tight-knit community. But beneath her infectious laughter lay a secret—a secret she had kept hidden from even those closest to her.

It started with a persistent cough—a nagging tickle in the back of her throat that refused to relent. At first, Maria brushed it off as nothing more than a minor inconvenience, a fleeting nuisance in the grand tapestry of life. But as the days turned into weeks and the cough persisted, a seed of doubt began to take root in her mind—a seed that whispered of darker truths lurking just beyond the horizon.

Reluctantly, Maria sought solace in the familiar halls of her neighborhood clinic—a place where healers and caregivers worked tirelessly to ease the burdens of those in need. It was here, amidst the sterile scent of antiseptic and the soft hum of fluorescent lights, that Maria's world would be forever changed.

The diagnosis came like a thunderclap—a deafening roar that shattered the tranquility of her existence and sent shockwaves rippling through the fabric of her reality. Lung cancer, they said—the words hung heavy in the air, suffocating her with their weight, choking her with their finality.

For Maria, the diagnosis was not just a medical term—it was a sentence, a verdict handed down by fate itself. It cast a shadow over her hopes and dreams, casting doubt upon the future she had once held so dear. But amidst the darkness, a flicker of determination ignited within her—a spark of resilience that refused to be extinguished.

Armed with courage and fortified by the unwavering support of her loved ones, Maria embarked on a journey—a journey into the heart of the unknown, where the path ahead was shrouded in mist and uncertainty. But with each step she took, Maria discovered a strength she never knew she possessed—a strength born from the depths of adversity, tempered by the fires of resilience, and forged in the crucible of her own indomitable spirit.

Along the way, Maria encountered others—kindred spirits whose lives had been touched by the same shadow that loomed over her own. There was Antonio, a retired factory worker whose lungs bore the scars of a lifetime spent toiling in the smog-choked air of the industrial heartland. And there was Sofia, a young mother whose world had been turned upside down by a diagnosis that threatened to tear her family apart.

But amidst the shared sorrow and collective struggle, there were moments of triumph—small victories won against the backdrop of adversity, each one a testament to the resilience of the human spirit. Together, Maria and her companions navigated the labyrinthine corridors of treatment and recovery, each step bringing them closer to the light at the end of the tunnel.

And so, dear reader, our story unfolds—a tale of courage in the face of uncertainty, of hope amidst despair, and of the enduring power of the human spirit to overcome even the greatest of challenges. It is a story that resonates with us all—a story of life, of love, and of the unbreakable bonds that unite us in our shared journey through the labyrinth of existence.

In the pages that follow, we will embark on a journey—a journey into the heart of lung cancer, where science meets compassion, where hope meets despair, and where the human spirit soars against the backdrop of adversity. It is a journey that will challenge us, inspire us, and ultimately, transform us in ways we never thought possible.

So join me, dear reader, as we embark on this odyssey together—a journey of discovery, of enlightenment, and of the unwavering belief that even in the darkest of nights, the light of hope still shines bright. For in the end, it is not the shadow that defines us, but the courage with which we face it—the indomitable spirit that burns within us, illuminating the path forward and guiding us towards a brighter tomorrow.

Chapter 1

Anatomy and Function of the Lungs

Prologue To Pulmonary Anatomy

The human respiratory framework is a wonder of natural designing, finely tuned to work with the trading of gases vital forever. At the core of this many-sided framework lie the lungs — two springy, cone-formed organs that act as the essential site of gas trade inside the body. In this section, we will leave on an excursion into the profundities of pneumonic life systems, investigating the construction and capability of the lungs in lovely detail.

**1.1 The Construction of the Respiratory System

The respiratory framework includes an intricate organization of organs, tissues, and designs committed to the trading of oxygen and carbon dioxide between the body and the outside climate. At its center are the lungs, which are isolated into two principal curves — the right lung and the left lung. Every lung is additionally partitioned into curves, with the right lung containing three curves (upper, center, and lower) and the left lung containing two curves (upper and lower).

Encompassing the lungs is a defensive film known as the pleura, which comprises of two layers — the instinctive pleura, which covers the outer layer of the lungs, and the parietal pleura, which lines the inward surface of the chest depression. The space between these two layers, known as the pleural cavity, contains a limited quantity of greasing up liquid that lessens rubbing during relaxing.

**1.2 The Life systems of the Lungs

Inside every lung, a stretching organization of aviation routes referred to as the bronchial tree fills in as the channel for air to make a trip to and from the alveoli — the minuscule air sacs where gas trade happens. The bronchial tree starts with the windpipe, or windpipe, which branches into the left and right fundamental bronchi. These primary bronchi further gap into more modest bronchi, bronchioles, and eventually, terminal bronchioles, which end in groups of alveoli.

The alveoli are the site of gas trade in the lungs, where oxygen from breathed in air diffuses across the flimsy walls of the alveoli and into the circulation system, while carbon dioxide — a side-effect of cell digestion — is ousted from the circulatory system and breathed out from the body.

**1.3 The Mechanics of Breathing

The course of breathing, otherwise called ventilation, is a unique exchange of solid withdrawals and changes in thoracic strain that work with the development of air into and out of the lungs. At the focal point of this cycle is the stomach — a vault molded muscle that isolates the chest cavity from the stomach cavity and assumes a critical part in the mechanics of relaxing.

During inward breath, the stomach contracts and levels, making the volume of the thoracic pit increment and the tension inside the lungs to diminish. This lessening in pressure makes a strain slope that brings air into the lungs through the open aviation routes. The intercostal muscles, arranged between the ribs, additionally aid this interaction by hoisting the ribcage, further growing the thoracic cavity.

On the other hand, during exhalation, the stomach and intercostal muscles unwind, permitting the versatile backlash of the lungs and chest wall to remove air. The multifaceted equilibrium of these strong activities guarantees a constant and cadenced trade of air, keeping a sensitive balance fundamental for supporting life.

**1.4 The Job of Surfactant

Inside the alveoli, a particular substance called surfactant assumes an essential part in lessening surface pressure and forestalling the breakdown of the little air sacs. Created by type II alveolar cells, surfactant is a combination of lipids and proteins that lines the alveolar surfaces. Its presence brings down the surface pressure of the liquid covering the alveoli, keeping them from imploding and working with the proficient trade of gases.

Understanding the job of surfactant is crucial, particularly with regards to respiratory misery disorder in babies, where deficient surfactant creation can prompt troubles in lung extension and compromised relaxing.

1.5 Vascular Stock to the Lungs

The lungs get a rich vascular stock to help the unpredictable course of gas trade. The pneumonic conduits, starting from the right half of the heart, convey deoxygenated blood to the lungs. Inside the pneumonic vessels encompassing the alveoli, carbon dioxide is delivered, and oxygen is consumed into the circulation system.

Oxygenated blood then, at that point, gets back to the left half of the heart through the aspiratory veins, fit to be siphoned into the fundamental course to feed the body's tissues and organs. This double circulatory pathway — the pneumonic dissemination for gas trade and the foundational flow for conveying oxygenated blood to the body — supports the respiratory and cardiovascular collaboration that supports life.

**1.6 Brain Guideline of Breathing

The multifaceted dance of breathing is coordinated by the respiratory focuses in the brainstem, explicitly the medulla oblongata and the pons. These focuses answer tactile contribution from chemoreceptors and mechanoreceptors, changing the rate and profundity of breathing to keep up with ideal degrees of oxygen and carbon dioxide in the blood.

Chemoreceptors delicate to changes in blood oxygen, carbon dioxide, and pH levels assume a crucial part in controlling relaxing. At the point when oxygen levels drop or carbon dioxide levels rise, signals from these receptors brief changes in the respiratory rate and profundity to reestablish harmony.

**1.7 Formative Considerations

Understanding the life structures and capability of the lungs additionally includes an investigation of their turn of events, from undeveloped stages to adulthood. The unpredictable course of lung advancement incorporates the development of the respiratory diverticulum, lung buds, and the development of different cell types that add to the perplexing engineering of the respiratory framework.

An enthusiasm for the formative excursion gives bits of knowledge into intrinsic circumstances influencing the respiratory framework and reveals insight into the weaknesses and versatility of the lungs at various phases of life.

**1.8 Normal Peculiarities and Variations

Likewise with any complex organic framework, varieties and abnormalities might happen in the life systems of the lungs. This segment dives into normal inherent peculiarities, like bronchial irregularities, lung agenesis, and varieties in location. Understanding these varieties is fundamental for medical services experts in diagnosing and overseeing respiratory circumstances actually.

1.9 Clinical Ramifications and Demonstrative Imaging

An extensive comprehension of pneumonic life systems is priceless in the clinical domain, particularly in the finding and the executives of respiratory problems. This segment investigates the use of analytic imaging procedures, like chest X-beams, figured tomography (CT) examines, and bronchoscopy, in envisioning the lungs and recognizing anomalies.

1.10 Conclusion: The Orchestra of Breath

As we finish up our excursion into the complex universe of pneumonic life structures, we feel overwhelmed by the ensemble of breath — an ensemble directed by the stomach, organized by the brainstem, and worked out in the sensitive dance of the lungs. The physical complexities and physiological wonders that empower every breath feature the stunning plan of the respiratory framework — a plan that supports life and interfaces us to the actual embodiment of our reality.

In the sections that follow, we will dig further into the subtleties of respiratory wellbeing and pathology, investigating the horde manners by which this multifaceted framework can be both tough and vulnerable. From the infinitesimal alveoli to the brain connections controlling breathing, the excursion proceeds — an excursion into the core of respiratory science, where every disclosure carries us closer to opening the secrets of the breath of life.

Chapter 2

Causes and Risk Factors

Understanding the etiology of cellular breakdown in the lungs includes exploring a complicated scene of joined factors, from natural openings to hereditary inclinations. In this part, we disentangle the diverse embroidered artwork of causes and hazard factors that add to the advancement of cellular breakdown in the lungs, revealing insight into the complex transaction between hereditary qualities, way of life decisions, and natural impacts.

**2.1 Tobacco Smoking and Lung Cancer

* **Verifiable Context:

  - The connection between tobacco smoking and cellular breakdown in the lungs was initial laid out during the twentieth hundred years through epidemiological examinations.

  - Top health spokesperson's Report: The critical 1964 report conclusively connected smoking to cellular breakdown in the lungs, molding general wellbeing arrangements.

* **Cancer-causing Components:

  - Tobacco smoke contains more than 7,000 synthetic substances, with no less than 250 distinguished as destructive and north of 60 perceived as cancer-causing agents.

  - Essential offenders: Polycyclic sweet-smelling hydrocarbons (PAHs), nitrosamines, and weighty metals.

* **Portion Reaction Relationship:

  - The gamble of cellular breakdown in the lungs increments with the span and force of smoking.

  - Smoking end: The gamble diminishes steadily subsequent to stopping, stressing the significance of smoking end programs.

* **Handed down Smoke:

  - Non-smokers presented to handed-down cigarette smoke additionally face a raised gamble of cellular breakdown in the lungs.

  - Approaches and mindfulness: Endeavors to lessen handed-down cigarette smoke openness in broad daylight spaces and homes.

**2.2 Word related and Ecological Exposures

* **Word related Hazards:

  - Asbestos Openness: Laborers in enterprises like development, shipbuilding, and protection are at expanded risk.

- Radon Openness: Radioactive gas saturating homes and work environments, particularly in specific land regions.

- Cancer-causing agents in the Work environment: Openness to cancer-causing substances like arsenic, chromium, and nickel in unambiguous businesses.

* **Ecological Factors:

- Air Contamination: Metropolitan regions with elevated degrees of air poisons add to cellular breakdown in the lungs risk.

- Indoor Air Quality: Openness to indoor poisons, for example, cooking vapor and biomass smoke, can likewise assume a part.

* **Radiation Exposure:

- Radon Gas: A main source of cellular breakdown in the lungs among non-smokers, frequently saturating homes starting from the earliest stage.

- Clinical Radiation: Total openness from analytic and restorative radiation.

**2.3 Hereditary Elements and Family History

* **Hereditary Predisposition:

- Familial Conglomeration: Presence of cellular breakdown in the lungs in various relatives recommends a hereditary part.

- Expansive Affiliation Studies (GWAS): Recognizing normal hereditary variations related with expanded cellular breakdown in the lungs risk.

* **Acquired Syndromes:

- Li-Fraumeni Condition: Germline changes in the TP53 quality increment helplessness to different diseases, including cellular breakdown in the lungs.

- Genetic Nonpolyposis Colorectal Disease (HNPCC): Connected to changes in DNA fix qualities, possibly affecting cellular breakdown in the lungs risk.

* **Sub-atomic Pathways:

- EGFR Transformations: Certain changes in the epidermal development factor receptor (EGFR) quality increment weakness to cellular breakdown in the lungs.

- KRAS Transformations: Connected to a subset of non-little cell cellular breakdowns in the lungs (NSCLC).

**2.4 Other Gamble Factors and Arising Research

* **Dietary Factors:

  - Cell reinforcements: Studies investigating the effect of cancer prevention agents, for example, nutrients C and E, on cellular breakdown in the lungs risk.

  - Carotenoids: Exploring the job of dietary carotenoids, tracked down in products of the soil, in forestalling cellular breakdown in the lungs.

* **Actual Activity:

  - Defensive Impacts: Arising research proposing a possible connection between customary active work and diminished cellular breakdown in the lungs risk.

  - Instruments: Investigation of the physiological components fundamental to the defensive impacts of activity.

* **Ongoing Lung Diseases:

  - Ongoing Obstructive Pneumonic Infection (COPD): Long haul irritation and harm to the aviation routes as a potential gamble factor.

- Interstitial Lung Illness: Relationship with an expanded gamble of cellular breakdown in the lungs.

* **Hormonal Factors:

- Chemical Substitution Treatment (HRT): The effect of HRT on cellular breakdown in the lungs risk, especially among postmenopausal ladies.

- Sex Chemicals: Investigating the expected impact of sex chemicals on cellular breakdown in the lungs improvement.

**2.5 Orientation and Age Disparities

* **Orientation Differences:

- Generally higher rates among men: Reflecting verifiable smoking examples.

- Evolving patterns: Rising occurrence in ladies because of expanded smoking predominance.

* **Age-related Patterns:

- Frequency and mortality patterns across age gatherings.

- The meaning old enough in cellular breakdown in the lungs forecast and treatment reaction.

**2.6 Financial Variables and Disparities

* **Financial Status (SES):

- Influence on admittance to medical care, smoking discontinuance assets, and ecological openings.

- Tending to differences: Procedures for lessening cellular breakdown in the lungs trouble in distraught populaces.

* **Geographic Disparities:

- Local varieties in cellular breakdown in the lungs rate and mortality.

- Admittance to medical services in rustic versus metropolitan regions.

**2.7 Conclusion Exploring the Mosaic of Hazard Factors

As we explore the complicated mosaic of causes and hazard factors for cellular breakdown in the lungs, obviously its etiology is a powerful exchange of hereditary, natural, and way of life impacts. This part fills in as an establishment for understanding the different gamble scene, making ready for ensuing investigations into counteraction, early recognition, and designated mediations in the sections that follow. As we continued looking for unwinding the intricacies of cellular breakdown in the lungs, the strings of causation structure an embroidery that stretches out a long way past the limits of individual decisions, venturing into the domains of hereditary qualities, climate, and cultural designs.

Chapter 3

Pathology and Staging

Understanding cellular breakdown in the lungs goes past its clinical show; it digs into the minuscule domain of obsessive elements and stretches out to organizing, a basic cycle that guides treatment choices and forecast. In this section, we set out on an itemized investigation of the unpredictable pathology of cellular breakdown in the lungs and the organizing frameworks that give a guide to clinicians in evaluating the degree of illness.

**3.1 Histological Kinds of Lung Cancer

* **Non-Little Cell Cellular breakdown in the lungs (NSCLC):

  - **Adenocarcinoma:

    - Starts in glandular cells covering the aviation routes.

    - Most normal histological sort, particularly in non-smokers.

    - Subtypes: Acinar, papillary, and lepidic.

  - **Squamous Cell Carcinoma:

    - Emerges from squamous epithelial cells in the bronchial aviation routes.

    - Firmly connected with smoking.

    - Frequently halfway found.

  - **Huge Cell Carcinoma:

- A heterogeneous class of undifferentiated NSCLC.

- Contains enormous, ineffectively separated cells.

- Will in general develop more rapidly than other NSCLC types.

* **Little Cell Cellular breakdown in the lungs (SCLC):

  - **Exemplary Little Cell Carcinoma:

  - Quickly developing neuroendocrine cancer.

  - Solid relationship with smoking.

  - Ordinarily midway found.

  - **Joined Little Cell Carcinoma:

  - Contains components of both little cell and non-little cell parts.

  - More uncommon however presents indicative and remedial difficulties.

* **Other Interesting Types:

  - **Carcinoid Tumors:

  - Slow-developing neuroendocrine growths.

- Seldom connected with smoking.

- Can begin in the focal or fringe lung.

- **Salivary Organ Tumors:**

- Unprecedented cancers emerging from salivary organ type cells.

- Happen in the bigger aviation routes.

- Adenoid cystic carcinoma is a model.

* **Forerunner Sores and Preinvasive Lesions:**

- **Lung Adenocarcinoma In Situ (AIS):**

- Restricted to the aviation route lining cells.

- Regularly presents as ground-glass opacities on imaging.

- Magnificent anticipation if carefully eliminated.

- **Squamous Dysplasia:**

- Forerunner to squamous cell carcinoma.

- Distinguished through bronchoscopic biopsy.

- Treatment might include reconnaissance or intercession.

3.2 Sub-atomic and Hereditary Features

* **EGFR Mutations:

  - **Frequency:

   - More normal in non-smokers and adenocarcinoma histology.

   - More common in East Asian populaces.

  - **Helpful Implications:**

   - Designated treatments like EGFR tyrosine kinase inhibitors (TKIs) like erlotinib and gefitinib.

   - Further developed results contrasted with regular chemotherapy.

* **ALK Rearrangements:

  - **Frequency:

   - More predominant in more youthful, non-smoking patients with adenocarcinoma.

  - **Restorative Implications:

   - Receptive to ALK inhibitors like crizotinib, ceritinib, and alectinib.

   - Designated treatment related with delayed movement free endurance.

* **ROS1 Rearrangements:

- **Frequency:

    - Distinguished in a little subset of lung adenocarcinomas.

  - **Helpful Implications**:

    - Receptive to ROS1 inhibitors, for example, crizotinib.

    - Progressing investigation into enhancing treatment techniques.

* **KRAS Mutations:

  - **Frequency:**

    - Normal in lung adenocarcinomas, particularly in smokers.

    - Related with an unfortunate visualization.

  - **Remedial Challenges**:

    - Absence of designated treatments straightforwardly repressing KRAS.

    - Research progressing to create powerful KRAS inhibitors.

* **PD-L1 Expression:

 - **Immunotherapy Biomarker:

   - Higher PD-L1 articulation related with expanded reaction to invulnerable designated spot inhibitors.

 - **Clinical Implications:

   - Guides the choice of patients for immunotherapy.

   - Separates patients in view of probability of reaction.

**3.3 Arranging of Lung Cancer

* **TNM Arranging System:

   - **Cancer (T):

   - Portrays the size and degree of the essential cancer.

   - Subcategories incorporate T1, T2, T3, and T4 in light of cancer size and attack.

   - **Hub (N):

   - Shows the contribution of provincial lymph hubs.

- Subcategories incorporate N0, N1, N2, and N3 in view of the number and area of impacted hubs.

   - **Metastasis (M):

   - Signifies the presence or nonappearance of far off metastases.

   - M0 implies no far off metastasis, while M1 demonstrates the presence of metastases.

* **Clinical versus Neurotic Staging:

  - **Clinical Staging:

   - Still up in the air through imaging, bronchoscopy, and other non-careful strategies.

   - Guides introductory treatment choices.

  - **Neurotic Staging:

   - Laid out through careful resection and assessment of the growth and encompassing tissues.

   - Gives a more exact evaluation of the cancer's qualities.

* **Organizing of Non-Little Cell Cellular breakdown in the lungs (NSCLC):

  - **Stage I:

- Restricted to the lung without lymph hub association.

    - T1-2, N0, M0.

    - Careful resection frequently therapeudic.

  - **Stage II:

    - Limited cancer with association of adjacent lymph hubs.

    - T1-2, N1, M0 or T3, N0, M0.

    - Careful resection might be trailed by adjuvant treatment.

  - **Stage IIIA:

    - Broad lymph hub contribution or growth intrusion into neighboring designs.

    - T1-3, N2, M0 or T3, N1-2, M0.

    - Therapy might include a medical procedure, chemotherapy, and radiation.

  - **Stage IIIB:

    - Further lymph hub inclusion or attack into basic designs.

    - T4, any N, M0 or any T, N3, M0.

- Therapy procedures might incorporate simultaneous chemoradiation.

  - **Stage IV:

    - Far off metastases.

    - Any T, any N, M1.

    - Treatment centers around fundamental treatments, including designated treatments and immunotherapy.

* **Arranging of Little Cell Cellular breakdown in the lungs (SCLC):

  - **Restricted Stage:

    - Bound to one lung and close by lymph hubs.

    - By and large more receptive to treatment.

  - **Broad Stage:

    - Spread past the lung and territorial lymph hubs.

    - Treated with foundational treatments.

    - Anticipation frequently less ideal.

* **Imaging Modalities in Staging:

  - **CT Scans:

- Fundamental for assessing the degree of the essential growth and lymph hub inclusion.

 - **Positron Outflow Tomography (PET) Scans:

- Evaluates metabolic action and helps in distinguishing far off metastases.

 - **MRI:

- Gives nitty gritty pictures, especially valuable for surveying cerebrum association.

 - **Bronchoscopy and Biopsy:

- Direct representation and tissue inspecting for obsessive affirmation.

* **Multidisciplinary Way to deal with Staging:

 - **Growth Boards:

- Multidisciplinary conversations including oncologists, specialists, radiologists, and pathologists.

- Cooperative decision-production for ideal treatment systems.

 - **Incorporation of Atomic and Hereditary Information:

- Atomic profiling to illuminate designated treatment choices.

- Customized treatment plans in view of hereditary modifications.

* **Prognostic Elements in Cellular breakdown in the lungs Staging:**

  - **Execution Status:**

- Measures the patient's capacity to perform everyday exercises.

- Influences treatment decisions and in general anticipation.

  - **Histology and Atomic Characteristics:**

- Different histological sorts and hereditary changes might impact results.

  - **Reaction to Treatment:**

- Surveying the viability of starting medicines guides resulting mediations.

- Assessment through imaging and clinical assessment.

* **Progressing Advances in Arranging Techniques:**

- **Fluid Biopsies:

   - Location of flowing growth DNA to evaluate hereditary changes and screen treatment reaction.

   - Potential for less obtrusive observing throughout treatment.

 - **High level Imaging Techniques:

   - Consolidation of cutting edge imaging advances for more exact organizing.

   - Investigation of man-made reasoning applications in radiology.

3.4 Difficulties and Discussions in Pathology and Staging

* **Growth Heterogeneity:

 - **Intra-tumoral Heterogeneity:

   - Inconstancy inside a similar growth.

   - Suggestions for biopsy precision and treatment reaction.

* **Examining Techniques:

 - **Biopsy Challenges:

- Trouble in getting adequate tissue for complete sub-atomic examination.

- Significance of picking suitable biopsy locales for exact organizing.

* **Arranging Limitations:

- **Imaging Limitations:

- Challenges in recognizing little metastases or minute lymph hub contribution.

- Progressing endeavors to upgrade imaging advancements.

* **Development of Organizing Systems:

- **Refreshes and Revisions:

- Occasional modifications to arranging frameworks in light of arising proof.

- Challenges in offsetting effortlessness with far reaching growth portrayal.

**3.5 Conclusion: Exploring the Scene of Pathology and Staging

In the complicated scene of cellular breakdown in the lungs, pathology and arranging act as essential navigational devices, directing clinicians through the intricacies of determination, visualization, and treatment arranging. From the minute assessment of histological sorts to the naturally visible evaluation of growth degree, each detail adds to a complete comprehension of the illness. As progressions keep on disentangling the hereditary underpinnings and refine arranging methods, this part makes way for the resulting investigation of therapy modalities and procedures in the continuous journey to further develop results for people confronting cellular breakdown in the lungs.

Chapter 4:

Symptoms and Diagnosis of Lung Cancer

Cellular breakdown in the lungs, frequently alluded to as the "quiet illness," may appear with unpretentious side effects or stay asymptomatic until cutting edge stages. Opportune acknowledgment and precise determination are principal for starting compelling intercessions. This section digs into the assorted range of side effects related with cellular breakdown in the lungs and investigates the symptomatic modalities utilized in disentangling the intricacy of this illness.

**4.1 Early Admonition Signs and Symptoms

* **Tireless Cough:

  - **Description:**

    - A hack that waits for in excess of half a month.

  - **Related Characteristics:

    - Might be dry or produce mucus.

    - Can deteriorate over the long run.

* **Brevity of Breath:

- **Description:

  - Trouble in breathing or pausing to rest.

 - **Related Characteristics:

  - Might be slow or unexpected beginning.

  - Frequently deteriorates with effort.

* **Chest Pain:

 - **Description:

  - Uneasiness or torment in the chest, shoulder, or back.

  - **Related Characteristics:

  - Might be sharp or hurting in nature.

  - Power can change.

* **Wheezing:

 - **Description:

  - Sharp whistling sound during relaxing.

  - **Related Characteristics:

  - Normal in aviation route deterrent.

  - Can be irregular or determined.

* **Unexplained Weight Loss:

- **Description:

    - Huge weight reduction without clear reason.

  - **Related Characteristics:

    - Frequently demonstrative of cutting edge sickness.

    - Might be joined by loss of hunger.

* **Fatigue:

  - **Description:

    - Relentless sensation of sleepiness or shortcoming.

  - **Related Characteristics:

    - Can be lopsided to movement level.

    - Slows down day to day working.

* **Hoarseness:

  - **Description:

    - Changes in voice tone or quality.

  - **Related Characteristics:

    - Aftereffect of nerve association or aviation route deterrent.

- May continue regardless of vocal rest.

* **Continuous Infections:

 - **Description:

   - Intermittent respiratory diseases.

 - **Related Characteristics:

   - Result from compromised safe capability.

   - Frequently found in certain subtypes, as squamous cell carcinoma.

**4.2 High level Side effects and Foundational Manifestations

* **Hemoptysis:

 - **Description:

   - Hacking up blood or horrendous sputum.

 - **Related Characteristics:

   - Can change from streaks to bigger sums.

   - Disturbing side effect requiring brief assessment.

* **Trouble Swallowing:

 - **Description:

- Dysphagia or uneasiness while gulping.

  - **Related Characteristics:

    - May result from cancer pressure or intrusion.

    - Can prompt unexpected weight reduction.

* **Enlarging of Neck or Face:

  - **Description:

    - Noticeable expanding in the neck or face.

  - **Related Characteristics:

    - Aftereffect of lymph hub contribution.

    - May cause facial lopsidedness or venous blockage.

* **Bone Pain:

  - **Description:

    - Throbbing or distress in bones, frequently the spine or ribs.

  - **Related Characteristics:

    - Demonstrates metastatic spread to bones.

    - Might be exacerbated by development.

* **Neurological Symptoms:

- **Description:

    - Cerebral pains, dazedness, or appendage shortcoming.

  - **Related Characteristics:

    - Result from metastases to the mind or spinal line.

    - Can appear as seizures or mental changes.

* **Jaundice:

  - **Description:

    - Yellowing of the skin and eyes.

  - **Related Characteristics:

    - Indication of liver association or check of the bile pipe.

    - Shows progressed sickness.

* **Clubbing of Fingers:

  - **Description:**

    - Bulbous augmentation of fingertips.

  - **Related Characteristics:

    - Connected to ongoing hypoxia.

- Found at times of non-little cell cellular breakdown in the lungs (NSCLC).

4.3 Symptomatic Modalities and Screening Approaches

* **Imaging Studies:

  - **Chest X-Ray:

    - **Purpose:

      - Introductory screening device.

      - Identifies anomalies in the lungs.

    - **Considerations:

      - Restricted responsiveness for little or beginning phase growths.

      - Frequently followed by further developed imaging.

  - **Figured Tomography (CT) Scan:

    - **Purpose:

      - Definite imaging of the lungs and encompassing designs.

      - Distinguishes size, area, and degree of growths.

- **Considerations:**

    - High responsiveness for recognizing lung irregularities.

    - Fundamental for organizing and treatment arranging.

* **Positron Emanation Tomography (PET) Scan:

  - **Purpose:

    - Assesses metabolic movement of tissues.

    - Evaluates spread of malignant growth past the lungs.

Bronchoscopy:

  - **Purpose:

    - Direct perception of the aviation routes utilizing an adaptable degree.

    - Takes into consideration tissue examining and biopsy.

  - **Considerations:

    - Gives admittance to focal and fringe injuries.

    - Can be joined with other indicative modalities like endobronchial ultrasound (EBUS).

* **Biopsy and Tissue Sampling:

 - **Fine Needle Yearning (FNA):

   - Negligibly intrusive strategy utilizing a slim needle to extricate tissue tests.

   - Frequently directed by imaging modalities like CT or ultrasound.

 - **Transbronchial Biopsy:

   - Tissue testing through the bronchoscope.

   - Helpful for sores available by means of the aviation routes.

 - **Thoracentesis:

   - Expulsion of liquid from the pleural space encompassing the lungs.

   - Analyze pleural radiations and get cytology tests.

* **Sputum Cytology:

 - **Purpose:

   - Assessment of sputum under a magnifying instrument for strange cells.

- Harmless screening device.

- **Considerations:

- Restricted awareness and explicitness.

- Frequently utilized related to imaging and other demonstrative tests.

* **Genomic Testing:

- **Purpose:

- Distinguishes explicit hereditary changes and biomarkers.

- Guides treatment choices, especially for designated treatments.

- **Considerations:

- Incorporates testing for EGFR, ALK, ROS1, and different transformations.

- May include cutting edge sequencing (NGS) for complete profiling.

* **Aspiratory Capability Tests (PFTs):

- **Purpose:

- Assesses lung capability and limit.

- Evaluates respiratory side effects and useful hindrance.

  - **Considerations:

  - Supportive in deciding gauge lung capability before medical procedure or different mediations.

  - Screens illness movement and reaction to treatment.

* **Screening Approaches:

  - **Low-Portion CT (LDCT) Screening:

  - Suggested for high-risk people, like long haul smokers.

  - Identifies lung knobs at an early, possibly treatable stage.

  - Considered a savvy approach for cellular breakdown in the lungs screening.

  - **Screening Guidelines:

  - Proposals from associations like the U.S. Preventive Administrations Team (USPSTF) and the American Malignant growth Society (ACS).

  - Accentuate shared decision-production among patients and medical care suppliers.

**4.4 Difficulties and Contemplations in Diagnosis

* **Covering Symptoms:

  - Cellular breakdown in the lungs side effects can copy those of other respiratory circumstances, prompting demonstrative difficulties.

  - Differential conclusion significant for precise appraisal and convenient intercession.

* **Admittance to Care:

  - Differences in admittance to medical care administrations and analytic assets.

  - Financial elements, geographic area, and protection inclusion impact demonstrative pathways.

* **Histological Variability:

  - Cellular breakdown in the lungs envelops different histological subtypes with novel highlights.

  - Exact grouping fundamental for treatment determination and anticipation.

* **Symptomatic Delays:

- Deferred acknowledgment of side effects and reference to experts add to indicative deferrals.

- Elevated mindfulness among medical care suppliers and the public fundamental for early location.

4.5 Integrative Methodologies and Multidisciplinary Collaboration

* **Cancer Boards:**

- Multidisciplinary discussions including oncologists, pulmonologists, radiologists, pathologists, and specialists.

- Work with cooperative independent direction and individualized treatment arranging.

* **Patient-Focused Care:**

- Enabling patients to effectively partake in their consideration and dynamic cycle.

- Giving training and backing all through the indicative excursion.

* **Accuracy Medicine:**

- Fitting treatment systems in view of sub-atomic and hereditary profiling.

- Further developing treatment results and limiting unfavorable impacts through designated treatments.

**4.6 Conclusion: Exploring the Symptomatic Odyssey

In the maze of cellular breakdown in the lungs determination, perceiving the early admonition signs are urgent to utilize a complete symptomatic methodology. From the underlying assessment of side effects to the unpredictable trap of imaging studies and tissue testing strategies, each step adds to disentangling the analytic riddle. As progressions keep on rethinking demonstrative standards and improve accuracy medication draws near, the excursion toward early recognition and customized care proclaims another period in the battle against cellular breakdown in the lungs. Through cooperative endeavors and relentless responsibility, clinicians and patients the same set out on an aggregate journey to overcome this imposing enemy and prepare for a future where cellular breakdown in the lungs is identified early, treated really, and at last won.

Chapter 5

Surgery in the Management of Lung Cancer

Medical procedure assumes an urgent part in the exhaustive administration of cellular breakdown in the lungs, offering a likely solution for limited sickness and adding to whitewashing and side effect help in specific high level cases. This part digs into the assorted parts of careful intercessions for cellular breakdown in the lungs, enveloping preoperative contemplations, different surgeries, postoperative consideration, and progressing headways that shape the scene of cellular breakdown in the lungs medical procedure.

**5.1 Preoperative Appraisal and Patient Selection

* **Patient Evaluation:

 - **Clinical History:

   - Thorough appraisal of patient history, including existing together ailments, earlier medical procedures, and prescription history.

- Distinguishing proof of chance variables and streamlining of comorbidities.

  - **Pneumonic Capability Tests (PFTs):

    - Assessment of standard lung capability to survey the patient's capacity to endure a medical procedure.

    - Spirometry, lung volumes, and dissemination limit estimations.

* **Imaging Studies:

  - **CT Scan:

    - Nitty gritty imaging of the chest to survey cancer attributes, area, and degree.

    - Fundamental for careful preparation and deciding resectability.

  - **PET Scan:

    - Surveying metabolic movement and recognizing far off metastases.

    - Supports organizing and direction in regards to a medical procedure.

* **Cardiovascular Evaluation:

- **Electrocardiogram (ECG) and Echocardiogram:**

   - Evaluating heart capability and recognizing expected cardiovascular dangers.

   - Fundamental for careful leeway and limiting perioperative complexities.

* **Lab Tests:**

  - **Blood Counts and Biochemistry:**

   - Distinguishing irregularities that might influence careful office.

   - Assessing hematological and biochemical boundaries.

* **Pneumonic Rehabilitation:**

  - **Purpose:**

   - Improving respiratory capability and in general wellness.

   - Working on postoperative results and decreasing entanglements.

  - **Components:**

   - Practice preparing, breathing activities, and schooling.

- Joint effort with respiratory specialists.

* **Smoking Cessation:

  - **Benefits:

    - Further developed lung capability and wound recuperating.

    - Decrease in postoperative difficulties.

  - **Interventions:

    - Smoking end projects and backing.

    - Preoperative guiding and inspiration.

**5.2 Surgeries for Lung Cancer

* **Lobectomy:

  - **Description:

    - Expulsion of a whole curve of the lung.

    - Standard methodology for beginning phase cellular breakdown in the lungs.

  - **Advantages:

    - Maximal cancer leeway.

    - Jelly a critical part of lung capability.

* **Segmentectomy:

- **Description:

   - Evacuation of a portion of the lung containing the cancer.

   - Reasonable for specific instances of more modest growths or compromised lung capability.

  - **Considerations**:

   - Offsetting growth freedom with conservation of lung tissue.

   - Proper for explicit subtypes and beginning phase injuries.

* **Wedge Resection**:

  - **Description:

   - Expulsion of a little, wedge-formed part of the lung containing the cancer.

   - Considered for fringe, little cancers in select cases.

  - **Advantages**:

   - Reasonable for patients with restricted pneumonic save.

   - Negligibly obtrusive methodology.

* **Pneumonectomy:

  - **Description:

    - Evacuation of a whole lung.

    - Held for cases with broad growth inclusion or halfway found cancers.

  - **Considerations:

    - Critical effect on aspiratory capability.

    - Cautious patient determination in view of generally wellbeing and aspiratory save.

* **Negligibly Obtrusive Approaches:

  - **Video-Helped Thoracoscopic Medical procedure (VATS):

    - Uses little cuts and a Thoracoscopic for representation.

    - Appropriate for chosen instances of lobectomy and segmentectomy.

    - Decreased postoperative torment and more limited emergency clinic stays.

  - **Automated Helped Surgery:

- Consolidates automated frameworks for upgraded accuracy and mobility.

- Works with complex methodology with further developed perception.

- Comparable advantages to Tanks regarding diminished dreariness.

**5.3 Intraoperative Contemplations and Techniques

* **Sentinel Lymph Hub Biopsy:

  - **Purpose:

- ID and biopsy of the sentinel lymph hub to evaluate for malignant growth spread.

- Helps guide the degree of lymph hub analysation.

  - **Technique:

- Infusion of a tracer around the cancer.

- ID and evacuation of the primary lymph node(s) that get seepage from the growth site.

* **Mediastinal Lymph Hub Dissection:

  - **Purpose:

- Extensive expulsion of lymph hubs in the mediastinum.

- Precise arranging and appraisal of nodal contribution.

- **Technique:

- Deliberate analyzation of lymph hub stations in light of physical milestones.

- Improves the precision of arranging and illuminates postoperative treatment choices.

* **Nerve-Saving Techniques:

- **Repetitive Laryngeal Nerve Preservation:

- Safeguards the repetitive laryngeal nerve during a medical procedure.

- Lessens the gamble of vocal line loss of motion and voice changes.

- **Phrenic Nerve Preservation:

- Jam the phrenic nerve to keep up with diaphragmatic capability.

- Limits respiratory inconveniences postoperatively.

* **Intraoperative Imaging:

- **Fluorescence-Directed Surgery:**

   - Consolidates fluorescent colors to improve perception of growths and lymph hubs.

   - Works with exact recognizable proof and evacuation of harmful tissue.

 - **Intraoperative CT or MRI:**

   - Constant imaging during a medical procedure for upgraded exactness.

   - Valuable in complex cases to evaluate growth edges and guide resection.

**5.4 Postoperative Consideration and Complications

* **Emergency unit Stay:**

 - **Indications:**

   - Subject to the degree of medical procedure and the patient's general wellbeing.

   - Pneumonectomy or complex systems might require ICU checking.

 - **Monitoring:**

   - Respiratory status, cardiovascular solidness, and torment control.

- Avoidance and early location of entanglements.

* **Torment Management:

  - **Multimodal Approach:

    - Uses a mix of analgesics, including narcotics and non-narcotics.

    - Epidural or patient-controlled absense of pain might be utilized.

  - **Early Mobilization:

    - Empowers ambulation and profound breathing activities.

    - Decreases the gamble of postoperative entanglements.

* **Respiratory Care:

  - **Motivator Spirometry:

    - Elevates profound breathing to forestall atelectasis and pneumonia.

    - Ordinary use to keep up with lung capability postoperatively.

  - **Chest Physiotherapy:

    - Helps with clearing aviation route emissions.

- Benefits patients with compromised respiratory capability.

* **Complications:

  - **Aspiratory Complications:

    - Atelectasis, pneumonia, and respiratory disappointment.

    - Tended to through forceful respiratory consideration and early preparation.

  - **Heart Complications:

    - Arrhythmias, myocardial dead tissue.

    - Checking and the executives of cardiovascular status.

  - **Postpneumonectomy Syndrome:

    - Mediastinal shift prompting pressure of the leftover lung.

    - Requires close checking and conceivable mediation.

* **Recovery and Follow-Up:

  - **Aspiratory Rehabilitation:

- Fundamental for advancing lung capability and actual prosperity.

- Consolidates exercise, training, and psychosocial support.

  - **Long haul Follow-Up:

- Reconnaissance for repeat and observing for late difficulties.

- Steady consideration to address postoperative changes and upgrade personal satisfaction.

**5.5 Advances in Careful Procedures and Technologies

* **Improved Recuperation After Medical procedure (Times) Protocols:

  - **Purpose:

- Upgrades perioperative consideration to speed up recuperation.

- Limits postoperative entanglements and emergency clinic stay.

  - **Components:

- Early ambulation, nourishment streamlining, and multimodal torment the board.

- Executed across the careful continuum.

***3D Printing and Careful Simulation:

  - **Application:

- Preoperative preparation through 3D-printed models of the patient's life systems.

- Careful reproduction for complex systems.

  - **Benefits:

- Upgraded accuracy and diminished intraoperative time.

- Works with schooling and preparing for specialists.

* **Picture Directed Navigation:

  - **Route Systems:

- Utilization of continuous imaging to direct careful instruments.

- Improves precision in finding growths and basic designs.

  - **Applications:

- Especially significant in negligibly obtrusive techniques and complex life systems.

* **Robot-Helped Surgery:

  - **Da Vinci Careful System:

    - Integrates mechanical arms constrained by the specialist.

    - Empowers exact developments in bound spaces.

  - **Benefits:

    - Upgraded mastery and perception.

    - Diminished obtrusiveness and more limited emergency clinic stays.

**5.6 Contemplations for Extraordinary Populations

* **Old Patients:

  - **Assessment:

    - Complete geriatric appraisal to assess in general wellbeing.

    - Thought of fragility, comorbidities, and mental capability.

- **Individualized Approaches:**

- Custom-made careful plans in view of patient-explicit variables.

- Accentuation on keeping up with personal satisfaction and limiting perioperative dangers.

* **High-Chance Patients**:

- **Definition:

- Patients with critical comorbidities or compromised useful status.

- May incorporate people with old age, cardiovascular illness, or respiratory split the difference.

- **Risk-Advantage Assessment:**

- Cautious assessment of possible advantages against perioperative dangers.

- May include elective treatment modalities in specific cases.

* **Pediatric Patients:**

- **Rare Occurrence:**

- Lung cancer is extremely rare in pediatric populations.

- Tumors often present as sarcomas or primary lung malignancies.

  - **Multidisciplinary Approach:

    - Involvement of pediatric surgeons, oncologists, and supportive care teams.

    - Individualized treatment plans considering growth and development.

**5.7 Conclusion: Navigating the Surgical Frontier in Lung Cancer

The landscape of lung cancer surgery is continually evolving, guided by innovations in technology, a deeper understanding of tumor biology, and a commitment to individualized patient care. From meticulous preoperative assessments to advancements in surgical techniques and postoperative rehabilitation, each facet of the surgical journey is tailored to optimize outcomes and enhance the quality of life for individuals facing lung cancer. As the field embraces novel technologies and embraces a multidisciplinary approach, the surgical frontier in lung cancer continues to be a beacon of hope, offering both curative interventions and palliative strategies in the relentless pursuit of conquering this formidable disease.

Chapter 6

Radiation therapy:

1. **Introduction to Radiation Therapy:

Radiation treatment, otherwise called radiotherapy, is a clinical therapy that uses high portions of radiation to target and kill malignant growth cells. It is a critical part of malignant growth treatment and can be utilized alone or related to a medical procedure or chemotherapy.

2. **Types of Radiation Therapy:

   - *Outer Pillar Radiation: This includes coordinating an engaged light emission from outside the body to the disease site.

   - *Inward Radiation (Brachytherapy): Radioactive sources are set straightforwardly inside or exceptionally near the growth.

3. **Radiation Treatment Planning:

   - *Simulation: Exact imaging and estimations are taken to decide the treatment region.

   - *Therapy Planning: The radiation oncology group fosters a point by point intend to convey the endorsed portion while limiting openness to sound tissues.

4. **Radiation Conveyance Techniques:

   - *Force Regulated Radiation Treatment (IMRT): Permits exact command over the power and state of the radiation radiates.

- ***Stereotactic Radiosurgery (SRS):** Exceptionally engaged radiation utilized for little, distinct growths.

- ***Proton Therapy**: Uses protons rather than photons, considering exact focusing with negligible harm to encompassing tissues.

5. ****Side Impacts and Management:****

- ***Intense Side Effects**: Quick responses, for example, weakness, skin changes, and sickness.

- ***Long haul Side Effects: It** Can incorporate harm to encompassing tissues and expected auxiliary malignant growths.

6. ****Patient Training and Support:**

- ***Illuminating Patients**: Clear correspondence about the treatment cycle, likely secondary effects, and assumptions is imperative.

- ***Support Services**: Giving assets like advising, support gatherings, and instructive materials to assist patients with adapting to the close to home and actual difficulties of radiation treatment.

7. ****Advancements in Radiation Therapy:**

- ***Picture Directed Radiation Treatment (IGRT)**: Constant imaging guarantees exact focusing on.

- ***Immunotherapy in Combination**: Joining radiation treatment with immunotherapy to upgrade the resistant framework's reaction to malignant growth cells.

- ***Radiation Oncology Research**: Progressing studies to further develop therapy adequacy and decrease aftereffects.

8. ****Quality Affirmation and Safety:**

- ***Dosimetry**: Precise estimation and computation of radiation dosages to guarantee the recommended portion is conveyed.

- ***Radiation Wellbeing Protocols**: Severe adherence to somewhere safe and secure rules to safeguard both patients and medical care experts.

In rundown, Section 6 of radiation treatment covers the essential parts of therapy arranging, conveyance strategies, secondary effects, patient training, mechanical headways, and security measures. Nonstop exploration and headways in this field add to working on the viability and wellbeing of radiation treatment in the continuous fight against the disease.

Chapter 7

Chemotherapy And Targeted Therapy

Chemotherapy is a crucial part of disease therapy, including the utilization of strong medications to target and kill quickly separating cells, including malignant growth cells. This part digs into the complexities of chemotherapy, investigating its instruments, types, aftereffects, and the advancing scene of customized chemotherapy.

1. Components of Activity:

Cell Cycle Interruption: Chemotherapy upsets the phone cycle by impeding DNA replication or forestalling cell division.

Apoptosis Enlistment: Certain medications trigger customized cell demise, urgent for dispensing with disease cells.

Angiogenesis Restraint: A few chemotherapeutic specialists repress vein development, obstructing cancer development.

2. Sorts of Chemotherapy:

Adjuvant Chemotherapy: Given after essential therapy to annihilate remaining disease cells.

Neoadjuvant Chemotherapy: Managed before a medical procedure to recoil growths and work with careful evacuation.

Palliative Chemotherapy: Expects to reduce side effects and work on the personal satisfaction in cutting edge malignant growth stages.

3. Normally Utilized Chemotherapeutic Specialists:

Alkylating Specialists: Models incorporate cyclophosphamide, which obstructs DNA replication.

Antimetabolites: Methotrexate slows down cell digestion by copying fundamental substances.

Topoisomerase Inhibitors: Medications like etoposide target proteins associated with DNA structure.

4. Aftereffects:

Hematological Issues: Chemotherapy frequently smothers bone marrow, prompting sickliness, leukopenia, and thrombocytopenia.

Gastrointestinal Pain: Sickness, heaving, and the runs are normal incidental effects.

Balding (Alopecia): Quickly partitioning hair follicle cells are impacted, causing impermanent going bald.

Immunosuppression: Chemotherapy debilitates the insusceptible framework, expanding weakness to contaminations.

5. Arising Patterns in Customized Chemotherapy:

Genomic Profiling: Fitting chemotherapy in view of the hereditary cosmetics of the cancer.

Immunotherapy Blends: Incorporating immunotherapeutic specialists with chemotherapy for improved treatment results.

Nanotechnology: Using nanoscale drug conveyance frameworks to upgrade drug focusing on and decrease incidental effects.

6. Difficulties and Future Bearings:

Drug Opposition: Continuous exploration intends to beat obstruction components created by malignant growth cells.

Designated Treatments: Progressions in recognizing explicit sub-atomic targets add to additional exact and powerful medicines.

Patient-Driven Approaches: Incorporating patient inclinations and values into treatment choices for a more comprehensive methodology.

This part gives a thorough comprehension of chemotherapy's multi-layered nature, underlining its job in disease treatment while recognizing the difficulties and promising roads for future turns of events.

Chapter 8

Immunotherapy

**Prologue to Immunotherapy:

Immunotherapy is a progressive way to deal with disease therapy that saddles the body's own invulnerable framework to perceive, assault, and obliterate malignant growth cells. Dissimilar to conventional therapies, for example, chemotherapy and radiation treatment, which straightforwardly target malignant growth cells, immunotherapy helps the body's regular safeguards to upgrade the invulnerable framework's capacity to battle disease.

**Kinds of Immunotherapy:

1. **Checkpoint Inhibitors:

   - *Mechanism: These medications block designated spots that keep safe cells from going after malignant growth cells, permitting the invulnerable framework to mount a more grounded reaction.

   - *Examples: Pembrolizumab, nivolumab.

2. **CAR-Lymphocyte Therapy:

- ***Mechanism**: Illusory Antigen Receptor Immune system microorganism treatment includes changing a patient's Lymphocytes outside the body to communicate receptors focusing on unambiguous malignant growth cells.

  - *Examples: Kymriah, Yescarta.

3. **Monoclonal Antibodies:**

  - ***Mechanism**: Research facility created antibodies tie to explicit proteins on disease cells, hailing them for obliteration by the safe framework.

  - *Examples: Rituximab, trastuzumab.

4. **Cytokines**:

  - ***Mechanism**: Interleukins and interferons are controlled to invigorate the invulnerable framework and improve its capacity to perceive and annihilate malignant growth cells.

  - *Examples: Interleukin-2, interferon-alpha.

5. **Cancer Vaccines**:

  - ***Mechanism**: Animate the resistant framework to perceive and go after malignant growth cells by introducing explicit antigens related with the cancer.

   - *Examples: Sipuleucel-T.

**Instruments of Action:

1. **Activation of T Cells:

   - *Acknowledgment of Malignant growth Cells: Immunotherapy assists Lymphocytes with distinguishing disease cells as strange and targets them for obliteration.

   - *Upgraded Insusceptible Response: Enacting and increasing White blood cells to reinforce the invulnerable framework's capacity to battle disease.

2. **Disruption of Resistant Evasion:

   - *Designated spot Inhibition: Obstructing proteins that repress resistant reaction, permitting Lymphocytes to target malignant growth cells really.

   - *Defeating Growth Resistance: Immunotherapy beats components utilized by disease cells to sidestep recognition and annihilation.

**Clinical Applications:

1. **Melanoma and Skin Cancers:

   - *Spearheading Success: Immunotherapy has
shown momentous adequacy in treating progressed
melanoma, essentially working on tolerant results.

   - *Designated spot Inhibitors: Specialists like
pembrolizumab and nivolumab have become
standard medicines.

2. **Lung Cancer:

   - *First-Line Treatment: Immunotherapy has
been incorporated into first-line treatments for
particular kinds of cellular breakdown in the lungs,
further developing in general endurance rates.

   - *Mix Therapies: Frequently utilized in blend
with chemotherapy or different immunotherapies.

3. **Hematologic Malignancies:

   - *Vehicle Lymphocyte Therapy: Especially
fruitful in treating specific kinds of leukemia and
lymphoma, exhibiting high reaction rates.

  - *Monoclonal Antibodies: Involved in the therapy of different blood diseases, focusing on unambiguous surface markers on malignant growth cells.

4. **Solid Cancer Applications:

  - *Extending Landscape: Progressing research investigates the viability of immunotherapy in different strong growths, including bosom, prostate, and ovarian tumors.

  - *Biomarker Identification: Distinguishing explicit biomarkers predicts patient reactions to immunotherapy.

**Difficulties and Side Effects:

1. **Autoimmune Reactions:

  - *Safe Related Unfavorable Occasions (irAEs): Accidental resistant reactions against sound tissues, requiring cautious checking and management.

  - *Organ-Explicit Toxicities: Antagonistic impacts on organs like the skin, gastrointestinal parcel, and endocrine framework.

2. **Response Heterogeneity**:

   - *Patient Variability: Immunotherapy reactions can fluctuate essentially among people, prompting difficulties in anticipating results.

   - *Biomarker Identification: Progressing endeavors to recognize prescient biomarkers to tailor treatment techniques.

Future Headways and Advancements:

1. **Combination Therapies**:

   - *Designated spot Inhibitor Combinations: Investigating the synergistic impacts of consolidating different designated spot inhibitors.

   - *Immunotherapy and Designated Therapies: Exploring the capability of consolidating immunotherapy with designated treatments for improved adequacy.

2. **Personalized Immunotherapy**:

   - *Biomarker-Based Approaches: Using explicit biomarkers to customize immunotherapy medicines in light of individual patient profiles.

- *Genomic Profiling: Distinguishing hereditary transformations and modifications impacting immunotherapy reactions.

3. **Overcoming Resistance:**

- *Understanding Mechanisms: Exploring and addressing instruments prompting protection from immunotherapy.

- *Remedial Strategies: Creating novel ways to deal with defeat obstruction and improve supported reactions.

Conclusion:

Immunotherapy addresses a change in outlook in disease therapy, offering a designated and strong methodology that takes advantage of the body's resistant framework to battle malignant growth. While challenges exist, progressing research and clinical headways keep on extending the applications and work on the adequacy of immunotherapy, giving desire to more solid and customized malignant growth treatments later on.

Chapter 9

Emerging Therapies and Clinical Trials

As the scene of cellular breakdown in the lungs treatment keeps on developing, the quest for creative treatments and novel treatment modalities stays vital. Section 9 investigates the domain of arising treatments and the job of clinical preliminaries in molding the fate of cellular breakdown in the lungs the board. From immunotherapy forward leaps to designated specialists and then some, this part enlightens the promising roads that hold potential for changing the treatment worldview.

**9.1 Immunotherapy Advancements

* **Resistant Designated spot Inhibitors (ICIs):

  - **Overview:

    - ICIs have changed the therapy of cellular breakdown in the lungs by releasing the body's safe framework against cancer cells.

    - Target modified cell passing protein 1 (PD-1), customized demise ligand 1 (PD-L1), and cytotoxic T-lymphocyte-related antigen 4 (CTLA-4).

  - **Clinical Trials:

    - Examine the viability of ICIs as monotherapy or in mix with different specialists across different cellular breakdown in the lungs subtypes.

    - Survey long haul endurance results and prescient biomarkers for treatment reaction.

* **Bispecific Antibodies:

  - **Mechanism:

    - Connect with two unique targets at the same time to upgrade resistant cell actuation and growth cell killing.

- Divert Immune system microorganisms to cancer cells with high explicitness and power.

- **Clinical Trials:

- Investigate the restorative capability of bispecific antibodies in cellular breakdown in the lungs, including bispecific Immune system microorganism engagers (Nibbles) and double liking retargeting antibodies (DARTs).

- Assess wellbeing, decency, and antitumor movement in beginning stage studies.

* **Illusory Antigen Receptor (Vehicle) Lymphocyte Therapy:

- **Approach:

- Hereditarily alter patient's Lymphocytes to communicate Vehicles focusing on cancer related antigens.

- Empower Immune system microorganisms to perceive and wipe out disease cells.

- **Clinical Trials:

- Research Vehicle Immune system microorganism treatment in cellular breakdown in the lungs, especially in hard-headed or backslid cases.

- Evaluate practicality, security profile, and potential for tough reactions.

9.2 Designated Treatments and Accuracy Medicine

* **EGFR Tyrosine Kinase Inhibitors (TKIs):**

  - **Evolution:**

    - First-line therapy for EGFR-changed cellular breakdown in the lungs.

    - Beat obstruction components and improve remedial adequacy.

  - **Clinical Trials:**

    - Assess cutting edge EGFR TKIs, blend procedures, and instruments to postpone or conquer obstruction.

    - Investigate treatment sequencing and ideal term of treatment.

* **ALK Inhibitors:**

  - **Advancements:**

- ALK inhibitors exhibit exceptional adequacy in ALK-positive cellular breakdown in the lungs.

- Conquer obstruction changes and further develop results.

  - **Clinical Trials:

- Examine novel ALK inhibitors, blend treatments, and procedures to moderate obstruction.

- Survey focal sensory system viability and wellbeing profiles.

* **ROS1 Inhibitors:

  - **Emergence:

- ROS1-designated treatments show guarantee in ROS1-revised cellular breakdown in the lungs.

- Accomplish tough reactions and ideal security profiles.

  - **Clinical Trials:

- Investigate cutting edge ROS1 inhibitors and mix draws near.

- Survey adequacy in treatment-credulous and recently treated patients.

**9.3 Mix Treatments and Synergistic Approaches

* **Immunotherapy Combinations:

  - **Rationale:

  - Consolidate ICIs with chemotherapy, designated specialists, or other immunotherapy.

  - Advance synergistic antitumor impacts and improve resistant reactions.

  - Address potential obstruction components and expand helpful effect.

  - **Clinical Trials:

  - Explore different immunotherapy mixes in cellular breakdown in the lungs, including double resistant designated spot barricade and immunotherapy in addition to chemotherapy.

  - Evaluate wellbeing, adequacy, and likely biomarkers for patient separation.

* **Designated Treatment Combinations:

  - **Strategy:

- Join different designated specialists to conquer obstruction and upgrade treatment reactions.

- Explore double focusing of pathways associated with disease development.

- **Clinical Trials:

- Investigate mixes of EGFR TKIs with other designated specialists, for example, MET inhibitors or hostile to ongoing treatments.

- Evaluate adequacy in defeating obstruction and postponing sickness movement.

* **Chemotherapy and Immunotherapy:**

- **Rationale:

- Joining chemotherapy with immunotherapy to potentiate antitumor invulnerable reactions.

- Profit by the immunomodulatory impacts of specific chemotherapeutic specialists.

- **Clinical Trials:

- Assess the security and viability of chemotherapy in addition to immunotherapy in different cellular breakdown in the lungs settings.

- Research ideal treatment regimens and sequencing.

**9.4 Accuracy Oncology and Fluid Biopsies

* **Cutting edge Sequencing (NGS):

 - **Application:

 - Complete genomic profiling to recognize targetable modifications and guide treatment choices.

 - Identifies genomic changes past normal driver transformations.

 - **Clinical Trials:

 - Investigate the utility of NGS in fitting therapy techniques in cellular breakdown in the lungs.

 - Survey influence on treatment results and patient endurance.

* **Fluid Biopsies:

 - **Advancements:

 - Painless location of circling growth DNA (ctDNA) and other biomarkers.

- Observing illness movement, treatment reaction, and development of opposition.

  - **Clinical Trials:

    - Research the clinical utility of fluid biopsies in directing treatment choices and foreseeing treatment reaction.

    - Evaluate concordance with tissue biopsies and constant observing capacities.

**9.5 Novel Medication Conveyance Systems

* **Nanoparticle-Based Therapies:

  - **Concept:

    - Use nanoparticles for designated drug conveyance to malignant growth cells.

    - Further develop drug bioavailability and lessen askew impacts.

  - **Clinical Trials:

    - Investigate nanoparticle-based definitions in cellular breakdown in the lungs treatment.

    - Survey security, bearableness, and possible upgrades in treatment viability.

* **Intratumoral Medication Delivery:

  - **Approach:

  - Direct organization of remedial specialists into cancer tissue.

  - Defeat fundamental obstructions and upgrade nearby treatment impacts.

  - **Clinical Trials:

  - Research intratumoral drug conveyance draws near, including injectable warehouses and implantable gadgets.

  - Evaluate attainability, security, and effect on treatment results.

**9.6 Difficulties and Contemplations in Arising Therapies

* **Obstruction Mechanisms:

  - **Overview:

  - Addressing the rise of protection from designated treatments and immunotherapy.

  - Recognizing novel systems to beat obtained obstruction.

  - **Clinical Trials:

- Research mix treatments and sequencing procedures to postpone or forestall opposition.

- Investigate versatile treatment approaches in view of developing growth profiles.

* **Biomarker Identification**:

  - **Challenge:

  - Recognizing powerful prescient biomarkers for treatment reaction.

  - Customizing treatment determination in view of patient-explicit sub-atomic profiles.

  - **Clinical Trials:

  - Investigate novel biomarkers and integrate them into clinical preliminary plans.

  - Evaluate the legitimacy and dependability of arising biomarkers.

9.7 Moral and Administrative Contemplations in Clinical Trials

* **Informed Assent and Patient Autonomy:**

  - **Principles:

  - Guaranteeing exhaustive informed assent processes for cooperation in clinical preliminaries.

- Regarding patient independence and guaranteeing comprehension of likely dangers and advantages.

  - **Administrative Compliance:

  - Adherence to moral principles and administrative necessities in preliminary lead.

  - Protecting patient freedoms and prosperity.

* **Fair Admittance to Clinical Trials:

  - **Challenge:

  - Addressing differences in admittance to clinical preliminaries.

  - Guaranteeing portrayal of assorted patient populaces in research.

  - **Strategies:

  - Executing effort projects to improve mindfulness.

  - Teaming up with local area associations to further develop access.

**9.8 Patient Support and Involvement

* **Patient-Focused Research:

- **Worldview Shift:

  - Embracing patient points of view in concentrate on plan and execution.

  - Perceiving the significance of patient-announced results.

 - **Collaboration:

  - Drawing in tolerant backing gatherings and consolidating patient contribution to direction.

  - Cultivating organizations for shared objectives in cellular breakdown in the lungs research.

9.9 Conclusion: Exploring the Skyline of Possibilities

In the steadily advancing scene of cellular breakdown in the lungs treatment, arising treatments and clinical preliminaries enlighten the skyline of conceivable outcomes. From pivotal immunotherapy progressions to accuracy oncology and imaginative medication conveyance frameworks, the parts of disclosure are nowhere near shut. As specialists, clinicians, and patients stand at the front of these spearheading attempts, the cooperative quest for information and development prepares for a future where cellular breakdown in the lungs becomes treatable, however conquerable. As the excursion unfurls, the commitment of customized and viable treatments calls, directing us toward a skyline where the weight of cellular breakdown in the lungs is continuously lifted, each forward leap in turn.

Chapter 10

Coping with Diagnosis and Treatment

Getting a cellular breakdown in the lungs determination is a life changing second that starts a complex close to home excursion. Chapter 10 dives into the multi-layered parts of adapting to the analysis and exploring the difficulties of treatment. From mental and close to home contemplations to viable procedures for taking care of oneself, this part gives a far reaching manual for patients, parental figures, and their encouraging groups of people.

10.1 Close to home Effect of Diagnosis

* **Shock and Denial:

  - **Starting Reaction:

    - Numerous people experience a feeling of shock and doubt after hearing the conclusion.

    - Forswearing might act as a mental guard instrument to adapt to the staggering reality.

  - **Adapting Strategies:

    - Empowering open correspondence with medical services suppliers.

    - Giving assets to mental help and guiding.

* **Dread and Anxiety:

  - **Causes:

    - Apprehension about the obscure, treatment aftereffects, and expected results.

- Nervousness about the effect on day to day existence, connections, and what's in store.

  - **Adapting Strategies:

    - Presenting care and unwinding methods.

    - Offering admittance to help gatherings and psychological well-being experts.

* **Despondency and Loss:

  - **Grasping Loss:

    - Patients might encounter a feeling of grieving for their past lifestyle.

    - Lamenting possible tentative arrangements and assumptions.

  - **Adapting Strategies:

    - Giving a stage to articulation of melancholy and feelings.

    - Offering assets for melancholy directing and support gatherings.

**10.2 Structure a Help System

* **Family and Friends:

- **Job of Support:**

  - Loved ones assume a critical part in offering close to home and pragmatic help.

  - Go about as a wellspring of solace, support, and friendship.

  - **Correspondence Strategies:**

  - Working with transparent correspondence inside the encouraging group of people.

  - Teaching loved ones about the patient's requirements and inclinations.

* **Support Groups:**

  - **Benefits:**

  - Interfacing with people confronting comparative difficulties.

  - Sharing encounters, bits of knowledge, and methods for dealing with hardship or stress.

  - **Facilitation:**

  - Giving data on nearby and online care groups.

  - Empowering support in bunch exercises and conversations.

* **Proficient Counseling:

 - **Psychological wellness Professionals:

  - Clinicians, guides, and social laborers can offer specific help.

  - Tending to personal difficulties, nervousness, and ways of dealing with stress.

 - **Accessibility:

  - Guaranteeing data about accessible emotional well-being assets.

  - Lessening shame related with looking for proficient directing.

**10.3 Speaking with Medical care Providers

* **Patient-Supplier Relationship:

 - **Importance:

  - Building a trusting and cooperative relationship with medical services suppliers.

  - Upgrading correspondence for informed direction.

 - **Compelling Communication:

- Empowering patients to voice their interests, clarify some pressing issues, and look for explanation.

- Working with ordinary and open discoursed about treatment plans and assumptions.

* **Second Opinions:

- **Enabling Patients:

- Educating patients about the choice regarding looking for second suppositions.

- Building up the significance of being effectively engaged with treatment choices.

- **Facilitation:

- Giving assets and direction on getting second feelings.

- Addressing concerns and questions connected with looking for extra clinical points of view.

**10.4 Survival methods During Treatment

* **Mind-Body Practices:

- **Integration:

- Integrating practices like reflection, yoga, and profound breathing activities.

- Advancing unwinding, stress decrease, and generally speaking prosperity.

- **Access and Education:

- Offering assets and classes on mind-body rehearses.

- Working with admittance to integrative medication administrations.

* **Actual Exercise:

- **Benefits:

- Upgrading physical and psychological well-being during and after treatment.

- Easing treatment-related secondary effects and exhaustion.

- **Adaptability:

- Suggesting custom-made practice plans in view of individual abilities.

- Giving assets to specific activity programs for malignant growth patients.

* **Healthful Support:

- **Job of Nutrition:

- Addressing nourishing requirements to help generally wellbeing and treatment resilience.

- Overseeing aftereffects like weight reduction, queasiness, and craving changes.

- **Dietary Guidance:

- Teaming up with nutritionists to foster customized dietary plans.

- Offering instructive materials on sustenance during disease treatment.

10.5 Monetary and Down to earth Considerations

* **Monetary Counseling:**

- **Exploring Costs:**

- Grasping the monetary ramifications of disease treatment.

- Giving admittance to monetary directing administrations.

- **Asset Allocation:**

- Associating patients with monetary help programs.

    - Offering data on protection inclusion and accessible assets.

* **Commonsense Help Services:

    - **Transportation Assistance:

    - Addressing difficulties connected with movement for treatment.

    - Planning transportation administrations or rideshare programs.

    - **Home Consideration Services:

    - Working with admittance to home consideration for people with explicit requirements.

    - Guaranteeing a steady and agreeable home climate.

**10.6 Tending to Treatment Side Effects

* **Side effect Management:

  - **Proactive Approach:

    - Giving data on potential treatment aftereffects.

- Enabling patients to expeditiously report and address side effects.

 - **Strong Care:

- Working together with side effect supervisory groups, including torment trained professionals and palliative consideration suppliers.

- Offering assets on side effect help and survival methods.

* **Weakness Management:

 - **Instructive Resources:

- Illuminating patients about malignant growth related weariness and its effect.

- Offering systems for overseeing weariness through rest and movement balance.

 - **Physical and Close to home Support:

- Prescribing exercise programs custom-made to individual energy levels.

- Incorporating mental help to address profound parts of weariness.

**10.7 Survivorship Care Planning*

* **Progress to Survivorship**:

  - **Grasping Survivorship:

    - Perceiving the progress from dynamic treatment to survivorship.

    - Tending to the novel necessities and difficulties looked by survivors.

  - **Extensive Survivorship Plans:

    - Creating individualized survivorship care plans.

    - Consolidating data on follow-up care, likely late impacts, and way of life suggestions.

**10.8 Supporting Caregivers

* **Job of Caregivers:

  - **Critical Contributions:

    - Recognizing the fundamental job guardians play in the patient's excursion.

    - Perceiving the close to home and viable obligations guardians shoulder.

  - **Break and Support:

    - Underscoring the significance of taking care of oneself for guardians.

- Offering break administrations and care groups explicitly intended for guardians.

10.9 End of-Life Contemplations and Palliative Care

* **Advance Consideration Planning:

 - **Inception of Conversations:

  - Working with conversations about finish of-life inclinations and objectives of care.

  - Empowering patients to communicate their desires in regards to clinical mediations.

 - **Documentation:

  - Helping patients in recording advance orders and inclinations.

  - Guaranteeing openness of advance consideration arranging archives.

* **Palliative Consideration Integration:

 - **Comprehensive Support:

  - Coordinating palliative consideration from the get-go in the treatment direction for far reaching support.

- Zeroing in on side effect the board, close to home prosperity, and personal satisfaction.

  - **Communication:

  - Working with transparent correspondence about the job of palliative consideration.

  - Addressing misguided judgments and accentuating its corresponding nature to healing medicines.

* **Hospice Care:

  - **Timing and Transition:

  - Perceiving when remedial medicines may at this point not be reasonable.

  - Working with the progress to hospice care for solace and personal satisfaction.

  - **Family Involvement:

  - Including relatives in conversations about hospice care.

  - Offering close to home help and assets for families during this progress.

**10.10 Social and Otherworldly Considerations

* **Social Competence:

- **Individualized Care:

    - Perceiving and regarding assorted social convictions and practices.

    - Fitting consideration intents to line up with social inclinations.

  - **Correspondence Strategies:

    - Empowering open exchange about social contemplations.

    - Preparing medical services suppliers in social capability to improve patient-focused care.

* **Profound Support:

  - **Job of Spirituality:

    - Recognizing the significance of profound prosperity in adapting to ailment.

    - Giving admittance to otherworldly help administrations and chaplaincy.

  - **Comprehensive Care:

    - Establishing a comprehensive climate that regards different profound convictions.

    - Offering assets for patients to investigate and communicate their otherworldliness.

**10.11 Engaging Patients through Education

* **Data Accessibility:

  - **Clear Communication:

    - Guaranteeing that data is conveyed in justifiable language.

    - Keeping away from clinical language and giving composed materials to reference.

  - **Asset Hubs:

    - Making unified centers for instructive assets on conclusion, treatment, and steady consideration.

    - Offering on the web stages and pieces of literature for simple access.

**Health Literacy:

  - **Promotion:

    - Promoting health literacy to empower patients in understanding medical information.

    - Conducting workshops on interpreting medical literature and navigating healthcare systems.

  - **Advocacy:

- Encouraging patient advocacy for access to reliable health information.

- Promoting awareness of reputable online resources and support organizations.

10.12 Resilience and Adaptive Coping Strategies

* **Resilience Building**:

  - **Skill Development:

    - Encouraging the development of resilience through coping skill acquisition.

    - Providing resources for resilience-building workshops and support groups.

  - **Psychosocial Support:

    - Integrating psychosocial support services to enhance coping mechanisms.

    - Fostering a sense of community and shared experiences.

* **Adaptive Coping Strategies**:

  - **Personalized Approaches:

    - Recognizing that coping strategies vary among individuals.

- Facilitating exploration of adaptive coping mechanisms based on personal preferences.

  - **Mindfulness and Acceptance:

  - Promoting mindfulness practices and acceptance-based strategies.

  - Emphasizing the importance of adapting to changing circumstances.

10.13 Monitoring Mental Health and Seeking Help

* **Mental Health Check-ins:

  - **Regular Assessment:

  - Incorporating routine mental health assessments into follow-up care.

  - Identifying early signs of distress or mental health challenges.

  - **Stigma Reduction:

  - Normalizing discussions about mental health and seeking help.

  - Educating patients about the availability of mental health services.

* **Professional Mental Health Support:

  - **Access and Availability:

  - Ensuring accessibility to mental health professionals.

  - Offering counseling services and psychiatric support as part of comprehensive care.

  - **Integration with Care Teams:

  - Collaborating with mental health professionals as integral members of the healthcare team.

  - Coordinating efforts to address both physical and mental health aspects.

**10.14 Empowering Patients to Advocate for Themselves

* **Self-Advocacy Skills:

  - **Education and Training:

  - Providing education on self-advocacy skills.

  - Conducting workshops on effective communication with healthcare providers.

  - **Resource Navigation:

- Equipping patients with tools to navigate healthcare systems and access support services.

    - Fostering a sense of empowerment in managing their own care.

* **Peer Advocacy:

  - **Support Networks:

    - Encouraging participation in patient advocacy groups.

    - Leveraging the power of peer support for collective advocacy efforts.

  - **Educational Campaigns:

    - Initiating campaigns to raise awareness about patient rights and advocacy.

    - Building a community of empowered patients advocating for improved care.

**10.15 Building Hope and Maintaining Positivity

* **Hope as a Coping Mechanism:

  - **Psychological Impact:

- Recognizing the role of hope in coping with illness.

- Understanding the dynamic nature of hope throughout the cancer journey.

- **Cultivating Hope:

- Integrating hope-building interventions into supportive care plans.

- Promoting activities and narratives that inspire and uplift.

* **Positive Psychology Practices:

- **Strength-Based Approach:**

- Incorporating positive psychology principles into supportive care.

- Identifying and building on individual strengths and resilience factors.

- **Gratitude and Mindset:**

- Encouraging gratitude practices and fostering a positive mindset.

- Integrating positive psychology interventions for mental well-being.

10.16 Conclusion: A Comprehensive Approach to Coping

In the face of a lung cancer diagnosis, coping involves a multidimensional approach that encompasses emotional, social, practical, and spiritual aspects. By addressing the diverse needs of patients and their support networks, healthcare providers can contribute to a more resilient and empowered community. This chapter serves as a guide to navigating the complexities of diagnosis and treatment, fostering a culture of support, and empowering individuals to navigate their unique cancer journey with strength, dignity, and a sense of agency.

Chapter 11

Lifestyle and Wellness

Living with cellular breakdown in the lungs includes different difficulties, including actual side effects, profound pain, and changes in day to day existence. Notwithstanding, embracing a sound way of life and zeroing in on health can essentially affect the general prosperity and personal satisfaction for cellular breakdown in the lungs patients. In this far reaching guide, we'll investigate the vital parts of way of life and health customized to help cellular breakdown in the lungs patients all through their excursion.

**1. Nourishment and Diet

Keeping a fair and nutritious eating regimen is vital for cellular breakdown in the lungs patients to help by and large wellbeing, energy levels, and safe capability. Here are a few dietary suggestions:

- **Smart dieting Patterns**: Underline an eating regimen wealthy in organic products, vegetables, entire grains, lean proteins, and solid fats. Go for the gold of bright foods grown from the ground to acquire fundamental nutrients, minerals, and cancer prevention agents.

- **Protein Intake**: Incorporate sufficient protein sources like poultry, fish, vegetables, nuts, seeds, and dairy items to help muscle strength, insusceptible capability, and tissue fix.

- **Hydration**: Stay very much hydrated by drinking a lot of water over the course of the day. Limit admission of sweet refreshments and liquor, as they can add to drying out and influence generally speaking wellbeing.

- **Supplementation**: Relying upon individual necessities and clinical guidance, think about supplementation with nutrients, minerals, or nourishing enhancements to address explicit lacks or backing treatment results.

- **Unique Considerations**: Patients going through specific therapies like chemotherapy or radiation treatment might encounter changes in taste, craving, or assimilation. Work with a medical services supplier or nutritionist to address these difficulties and adjust dietary decisions in like manner.

**2. Actual work and Exercise

Ordinary actual work and exercise assume an essential part in working on generally speaking wellness, overseeing side effects, and improving personal satisfaction for cellular breakdown in the lungs patients. Here are some activity rules:

- **Consultation: Prior to beginning any activity program, talk with your medical care group to survey your wellness level, ailment, and any possible impediments or safety measures.

- **Kinds of Exercise: Consolidate a blend of high-impact works out (e.g., strolling, cycling, swimming) to work on cardiovascular wellbeing, strength preparing (e.g., weightlifting, obstruction groups) to develop muscle fortitude, and adaptability works out (e.g., extending, yoga) to improve versatility and decrease solidness.

- **Steady Progression: Start with low-influence exercises and bit by bit increment power, term, and recurrence in view of your resilience and solace level. Pay attention to your body and abstain from propelling yourself excessively hard, particularly during treatment or recuperation periods.

- **Adaptations: Relying upon treatment aftereffects or actual constraints, change work-out schedules on a case by case basis. Center around delicate developments, breathing strategies, and versatile activities to oblige changes in energy levels or portability.

- **Security Precautions: Focus on wellbeing safety measures like legitimate warm-up and chill off schedules, hydration, wearing fitting dress and footwear, and staying away from high-risk exercises that might present injury gambles.

3. Close to home Prosperity and Mental Health

Adapting to cellular breakdown in the lungs includes tending to personal difficulties, overseeing pressure, and supporting mental prosperity. Here are methodologies for everyday reassurance and psychological well-being:

- **Close to home Expression: Permit yourself to communicate a scope of feelings, including trouble, dread, outrage, and vulnerability. Look for source for profound articulation through journaling, conversing with a confided in companion or guide, or partaking in help gatherings.

- **Care and Unwinding Techniques: Practice care contemplation, profound breathing activities, moderate muscle unwinding, or directed symbolism to advance unwinding, lessen uneasiness, and upgrade close to home flexibility.

- **Stress Management: Distinguish stressors in your day to day existence and foster techniques to actually oversee pressure. This might incorporate time usage procedures, focusing on errands, defining limits, and participating in pressure decreasing exercises like leisure activities, imaginative outlets, or nature strolls.

- **Social Support: Develop major areas of strength for an organization of companions, relatives, support gatherings, or psychological well-being experts who can give sympathy, consolation, and functional help during testing times.

- **Proficient Counseling: Think about looking for proficient directing or treatment to address profound misery, survival techniques, and acclimation to life changes related with cellular breakdown in the lungs determination and treatment.

**4. Rest Quality and Supportive Rest

Quality rest is fundamental for generally wellbeing, safe capability, and recuperation during cellular breakdown in the lungs treatment. Here are ways to further develop rest quality:

- **Rest Hygiene: Lay out a reliable rest plan with customary sleep time and wake-up times. Make a loosening up sleep time schedule that incorporates exercises like perusing, paying attention to quieting music, or cleaning up to indicate to your body that now is the ideal time to rest.

- **Agreeable Rest Environment: Establish an agreeable rest climate that is dim, tranquil, cool, and liberated from interruptions. Utilize happy with bedding, pads, and beddings that help supportive rest.

- **Limit Stimulants: Stay away from energizers like caffeine, nicotine, and electronic gadgets near sleep time, as they can impede rest quality and upset the rest wake cycle.

- **Mind-Body Relaxation: Practice unwinding procedures before sleep time, like delicate extending, moderate muscle unwinding, or reflection, to advance unwinding and set up your body for rest.

- **Tending to Rest Issues: On the off chance that you experience steady rest issues like a sleeping disorder, rest apnea, or fretful legs condition, examine them with your medical care supplier for assessment and suitable administration.

**5. Smoking End and Tobacco Control

For cellular breakdown in the lungs patients who smoke or use tobacco items, stopping smoking is a basic move toward further developing treatment results, diminishing difficulties, and upgrading generally speaking wellbeing. Here are methodologies for smoking suspension and tobacco control:

- **Smoking End Programs: Look for help from smoking suspension programs, guiding administrations, or medical services suppliers represented considerable authority in tobacco discontinuance. These projects offer customized systems, conduct intercessions, and nicotine substitution treatments to assist you with stopping smoking.

- **Nicotine Substitution Therapy: Think about utilizing nicotine substitution items like patches, gums, capsules, or physician recommended prescriptions to oversee nicotine withdrawal side effects and desires during the stopping system.

- **Conduct Support: Consolidate nicotine supplanting treatment with social help, directing, or support gatherings to address mental parts of tobacco enslavement, foster adapting abilities, and forestall backslide.

- **Way of life Changes: Embrace sound way of life changes that help smoking end, like expanding actual work, rehearsing pressure decrease strategies, further developing sustenance, and staying away from triggers or circumstances related with smoking.

- **Family and Social Support: Include relatives, companions, or encouraging groups of people in your quit-smoking excursion. Impart your objectives, look for consolation, and lay out a sans smoke climate to help long haul achievement.

**6. Correlative and Integrative Therapies

Correlative and integrative treatments can supplement ordinary clinical therapies and advance comprehensive prosperity for cellular breakdown in the lungs patients. Here are a few integral ways to deal with consider:

- **Acupuncture: Needle therapy might assist with lightening side effects like torment, sickness, weariness, and nervousness. Talk with a certified acupuncturist experienced in working with malignant growth patients for protected and compelling medicines.

- **Knead Therapy: Back rub treatment can give unwinding, help with discomfort, stress decrease, and worked on personal satisfaction for cellular breakdown in the lungs patients. Pick an authorized back rub advisor prepared in oncology knead for particular consideration.

- **Mind-Body Practices: Investigate mind-body practices like yoga, judo, qigong, or directed symbolism to advance unwinding, care, and close to home prosperity. Take part in classes or projects custom fitted to disease patients' necessities.

- **Natural Supplements: Exercise alert with home grown supplements and talk with a medical services supplier or integrative medication expert prior to utilizing home grown supplements. A few spices might collaborate with disease medicines or prescriptions, so guaranteeing wellbeing and efficacy is fundamental.

- **Nourishing Supplements: Examine with your medical care group about integrating wholesome enhancements like nutrients, minerals, cell reinforcements, or natural cures into your therapy plan. Guarantee that enhancements are protected, proof based, and viable with your general wellbeing and clinical medicines.

- **Care Based Pressure Decrease (MBSR): Consider taking part in care based pressure decrease programs that join care contemplation, delicate yoga, and mental social strategies. MBSR can assist with decreasing pressure, further develop adapting abilities, and improve generally prosperity.

- **Craftsmanship Treatment and Imaginative Expression: Take part in workmanship treatment, music treatment, or inventive articulation exercises as source for close to home articulation, unwinding, and self-disclosure. Investigate craftsmanship classes, studios, or online assets custom fitted to malignant growth patients.

*7. Monetary and Pragmatic Support

Managing the monetary and pragmatic parts of cellular breakdown in the lungs treatment can overpower. Here are techniques and assets to assist with overseeing monetary difficulties:

- **Protection Coverage: Audit your health care coverage inclusion, including benefits, copayments, deductibles, and inclusion for disease medicines, prescriptions, and strong consideration administrations. Comprehend your privileges and choices under your protection plan.

- **Monetary Counseling: Look for help from monetary advocates or social laborers who can give direction on exploring medical services costs, protection claims, monetary help programs, and monetary preparation during malignant growth therapy.

- **Patient Help Programs: Investigate patient help programs presented by drug organizations, not-for-profit associations, government offices, and malignant growth habitats. These projects might give monetary guide, medicine help, transportation administrations, or housing support for qualified patients.

- **Local area Resources: Use people group assets, magnanimous associations, malignant growth support gatherings, and promotion bunches that offer monetary guide, transportation administrations, lodging help, dinner conveyance, and other functional help for disease patients and their families.

- **Business and Work Accommodations: Speak with your boss about your malignant growth analysis, therapy plan, and any required work facilities or clinical leave. Comprehend your privileges under the Family and Clinical Leave Act (FMLA) and inability regulations, and investigate work environment facilities that help your wellbeing and prosperity.

**8. Social and Close to home Support

Exploring the profound and social effect of cellular breakdown in the lungs needs help from friends and family, companions, and medical services experts. Here are systems for getting to social and daily reassurance:

- **Steady Relationships: Develop strong associations with relatives, companions, guardians, and medical services suppliers who can offer compassion, support, and useful help all through your malignant growth venture.

- **Support Groups: Join disease support gatherings, online networks, or neighborhood associations that offer close to home help, data sharing, and companion associations with other cellular breakdown in the lungs patients, survivors, and guardians. Partake in help bunch gatherings, conversations, and instructive meetings.

- **Proficient Counseling: Think about individual guiding, psychotherapy, or psychological wellness administrations to address personal difficulties, survival methods, change issues, and stress the executives. Work with authorized specialists or advocates experienced in oncology and strong consideration.

- **Profound and Close to home Well-Being: Investigate otherworldly practices, care exercises, contemplation, petition, or unwinding procedures that advance otherworldly and profound prosperity. Interface with clerics, profound guides, or peaceful consideration administrations for extra help.

- **Expressive Expressions Therapies: Participate in expressive expressions treatments like workmanship treatment, music treatment, dance development treatment, or composing treatment to communicate feelings, process encounters, and advance recuperating and self-articulation.

**9. Palliative Consideration and Side effect Management

Palliative consideration centers around alleviating side effects, overseeing aftereffects, working on personal satisfaction, and tending to the comprehensive necessities of cellular breakdown in the lungs patients. Here are techniques for palliative consideration and side effect the board:

- **Side effect Assessment: Routinely survey and convey about your side effects, aftereffects, torment levels, and personal satisfaction with your medical services group. Be proactive in talking about side effect the executives methodologies and treatment objectives.

- **Multidisciplinary Approach: Work with a multidisciplinary group of medical services suppliers, including oncologists, palliative consideration trained professionals, torment the executives specialists, medical attendants, social laborers, and specialists. Work together on customized care designs that address physical, close to home, social, and profound parts of care.

- **Torment Management: Investigate torment the executives choices like prescriptions, non-pharmacological mediations (e.g., needle therapy, rub treatment, active recuperation), unwinding methods, and mental help to lighten torment and further develop solace.

- **Side effect Control: Address normal side effects and symptoms of cellular breakdown in the lungs and its medicines, for example, weakness, sickness, windedness, hunger changes, rest aggravations, tension, wretchedness, and mental changes. Execute side effect the executives techniques custom-made to your singular necessities.

- **Advance Consideration Planning: Talk about advance consideration arranging, treatment inclinations, and objectives of care with your medical services intermediary, relatives, and medical care suppliers. Consider making advance orders, living wills, and solid legal authority records to direct future medical care choices.

**10. Survivorship and Follow-Up Care

Survivorship starts from the snapshot of conclusion and go on all through the disease venture, zeroing in on recuperation, wellbeing, and long haul follow-up care. Here are methodologies for survivorship and follow-up care:

- **Survivorship Care Plan: Work with your medical services group to foster a survivorship care plan that layouts post-therapy follow-up care, observing timetables, suggested screenings, likely late impacts, survivorship assets, and wellbeing methodologies.

- **Observing and Surveillance: Go to standard subsequent arrangements, screenings, imaging tests, research center tests, and wellbeing evaluations as suggested by your medical services suppliers. Remain careful in observing for any indications of malignant growth repeat, new side effects, or wellbeing changes.

- **Wellbeing Promotion: Embrace wellbeing advancing ways of behaving and way of life decisions that help long haul prosperity, for example, keeping a sound eating routine, remaining genuinely dynamic, staying away from tobacco and liquor use, overseeing pressure, getting customary rest, and rehearsing taking care of oneself.

- **Close to home Adjustment: Acclimating to life after cellular breakdown in the lungs treatment includes profound and mental variation. Show restraint toward yourself, recognize your excursion, commend achievements, and look for help from survivorship programs, guiding administrations, or companion support gatherings.

- **Late Impacts Management: Know about likely late impacts or long haul results of disease medicines, for example, exhaustion, mental changes, lymphedema, neuropathy, cardiovascular dangers, richness concerns, and personal difficulties. Talk about methodologies for overseeing late impacts with your medical services group.

- **Health and Lifestyle: Spotlight on all encompassing wellbeing by focusing on taking care of oneself exercises, social associations, significant exercises, side interests, imaginative pursuits, and stress-easing rehearses. Participate in survivorship programs, instructive assets, and local area occasions that advance survivorship and prosperity.

**Conclusion

Way of life and health assume fundamental parts in supporting cellular breakdown in the lungs patients all through their excursion, from determination and treatment to survivorship and long haul prosperity. By taking on solid way of life propensities, getting to strong assets, overseeing side effects, supporting profound prosperity, and participating in survivorship care, patients can upgrade their personal satisfaction, strength, and in general wellbeing results. Team up with medical care suppliers, investigate steady administrations, and enable yourself to pursue informed decisions that advance wellbeing and recuperation.

This thorough aide gives a guide to integrating way of life and health systems into the consideration and the board of cellular breakdown in the lungs, advancing all encompassing prosperity and strengthening for patients, guardians, and medical care groups. Embrace the journey of survivorship, focus on taking care of oneself, and flourish in life past cellular breakdown in the lungs.

Chapter 12

Survivorship and Follow-Up Care

Survivorship: Embracing Life Past Lung Cancer

Envision the second when the specialist expressed those life changing words: "You have cellular breakdown in the lungs." It seemed like the ground underneath you disappeared, and a staggering rush of dread, vulnerability, and skepticism overwhelmed your being. In any case, you are a champion, a contender, and you chose to defy this imposing enemy head-on.

Quick forward to now. You've finished your therapy process — a tornado of chemotherapy meetings, radiation therapies, and surgeries. The street was unpleasant, fixed with difficulties, misfortunes, and snapshots of hopelessness. However, in the midst of the tempest, you found repositories of solidarity, strength, and fortitude you never knew existed inside you.

Presently, as you stand on the limit of survivorship, another part unfurls — one of trust, recuperating, and restoration. Survivorship isn't just about getting by; it's tied in with flourishing, embracing existence with restored life, and outlining a course towards health and prosperity.

The Survivorship Care Plan: Exploring the Street Ahead

Your oncologist gives you a record that feels like a guide — a survivorship care plan customized to direct you through the post-treatment stage. This thorough arrangement frames a guide for follow-up care, checking plans, suggested screenings, possible late impacts, survivorship assets, and health systems. It's your plan for exploring the street ahead with certainty and lucidity.

Observing and Reconnaissance: Cautiousness as a Companion

Standard subsequent arrangements become a foundation of your survivorship process. These visits are not just about clinical appraisals; they are snapshots of consolation, approval, and organization with your medical services group. You determinedly go to screenings, imaging tests, lab assessments, and wellbeing evaluations as suggested by your medical care suppliers. Watchfulness turns into your believed sidekick, enabling you to remain receptive to any indications of disease repeat, new side effects, or wellbeing changes.

Wellbeing Advancement: Developing Health from Within

Survivorship isn't just about overseeing disease; it's tied in with advancing all encompassing health and embracing a way of life that supports your psyche, body, and soul. You set out on an excursion of wellbeing advancement, focusing on taking care of oneself exercises, social associations, significant pursuits, and stress-easing rehearses.

- **Sound Eating: You embrace a fair and nutritious eating routine, wealthy in natural products, vegetables, entire grains, lean proteins, and solid fats. You enjoy the kinds of feeding food sources that fuel your body and backing your resistant framework.

- **Actual Activity: Exercise turns into your partner in wellbeing, as you participate in standard actual work customized to your wellness level and inclinations. Whether it's strolling in nature, rehearsing yoga, swimming, or moving, development turns into a festival of solidarity and imperativeness.

- **Stress Management: Stress-lessening strategies like care reflection, profound breathing activities, moderate muscle unwinding, and innovative articulation become piece of your everyday daily schedule. You develop versatility, internal harmony, and profound prosperity.

- **Rest Hygiene: Focusing on helpful rest turns into a non-debatable part of your wellbeing process. You establish a relieving rest climate, practice unwinding customs before sleep time, and honor your body's requirement for reviving rest.

- **Smoking Cessation: In the event that you were a smoker before your determination, you made the valiant stride of stopping smoking, realizing that it is one of the most significant activities for your drawn out wellbeing and prosperity.

Profound Change: Sustaining Brain and Heart

The close to home scene of survivorship is mind boggling — an embroidery woven with snapshots of euphoria, appreciation, strength, and intermittent influxes of dread or vulnerability. You recognize the close to home effect of your disease process and permit yourself space for mending, reflection, and development.

- **Observing Milestones: Every achievement in your survivorship process turns into a festival — a demonstration of your solidarity, fortitude, and perseverance. You mark commemorations, treatment achievements, and snapshots of appreciation for life's valuable gifts.

- **Looking for Support: You rest on the mainstays of help that encompass you — family, companions, parental figures, individual survivors, and medical care experts. You participate in help gatherings, guiding meetings, or profound practices that sustain your close to home prosperity.

- **Investigating Meaning and Purpose: Survivorship welcomes contemplation — an excursion of finding significance, reason, and versatility notwithstanding difficulty. You participate in exercises that give pleasure, satisfaction, and a feeling of direction to your life.

Overseeing Late Impacts: Exploring New Terrain

While malignant growth treatment brought mending, it likewise left — a scene of possible late impacts or long haul incidental effects. You stay careful, working intimately with your medical services group to address any late impacts that might emerge, like weakness, mental changes, neuropathy, cardiovascular dangers, or personal difficulties.

- **Side effect Management: You proactively oversee side effects, look for proper mediations, and take on survival techniques custom fitted to your singular necessities. Whether it's pain management techniques, restoration treatments, or psychosocial support, you focus on your prosperity.

- **Long haul Follow-Up: Normal subsequent consideration stretches out past clinical appraisals; it's about all encompassing prosperity. You take part in survivorship programs, instructive assets, and local area occasions that proposes backing, schooling, and association with individual survivors.

Wellbeing And Way of life: Flourishing in Life After Cancer

As you embrace life after disease, you rethink what health and way of life mean to you. It's not just about actual wellbeing; it's tied in with embracing a comprehensive way to deal with wellbeing that envelops brain, body, and soul.

- **Taking care of oneself Rituals: You focus on taking care of oneself ceremonies that renew your energy and support your spirit. Whether it's enjoying a mitigating shower, rehearsing fragrance based treatment, journaling your contemplations, or investing energy in nature, taking care of oneself turns into a non-debatable part of your everyday existence.

- **Care and Gratitude: Care rehearses extend your association with the current second, cultivating a feeling of quiet, clearness, and appreciation. You enjoy basic delights, develop appreciation for life's favors, and track down magnificence in snapshots of tranquility and reflection.

- **Significant Connections: Connections take on new importance as you esteem minutes with friends and family, develop significant associations, and develop sympathy, empathy, and consideration in your collaborations. You track down comfort and strength in shared encounters and steady organizations.

- **Individual Growth: Survivorship turns into an impetus for self-improvement and change. You embrace potential open doors for learning, investigation, and self-revelation. Whether it's chasing after new side interests, acquiring new abilities, or leaving on inventive undertakings, you embrace life's prospects with interest and energy.

Palliative Consideration and Steady Services

In your survivorship process, palliative consideration and strong administrations assume a significant part in upgrading your personal satisfaction, overseeing side effects, and tending to all encompassing necessities.

- **Palliative Care: Palliative consideration keeps on being a foundation of your consideration, zeroing in on easing side effects, overseeing incidental effects, further developing solace, and supporting your general wellbeing. You work together with a multidisciplinary group of medical services suppliers who design care plans to your one of a kind necessities and inclinations.

- **Steady Services: You access a scope of strong administrations that supplement your clinical consideration, including dietary guiding, pain management,restoration treatments, integrative medication, psychological wellness administrations, other worldly consideration, and social work support. These administrations engage you to explore difficulties, upgrade flexibility, and enhance your survivorship experience.

Promotion And Empowerment

As a cellular breakdown in the lungs survivor, you become a backer — a voice for mindfulness, schooling, and strengthening. You share your excursion, bring issues to light about cellular breakdown in the lungs, advocate for exploration, and backing drives that advance early discovery, admittance to quality consideration, and further developed results for all disease patients.

- **Instructive Outreach: You take part in instructive effort programs, public talking commitment, and backing drives that bring issues to light about cellular breakdown in the lungs risk factors, counteraction methodologies, screening rules, treatment choices, survivorship care, and strong assets.

- **Local area Engagement: You draw in with backing associations, malignant growth support gatherings, survivorship organizations, and local area occasions that enable patients, guardians, and medical care experts. You add to a steady local area that cultivates cooperation, sympathy, and strengthening.

- **Strategy Advocacy: You advocate for strategy changes, research financing, medical services access, and evenhanded consideration for cellular breakdown in the lungs patients. You speak more loudly to address variations, further develop medical services frameworks, and backer for approaches that focus on quiet focused care, survivorship support, and imaginative therapies.

Conclusion: Flourishing Past Cancer

In the embroidery of survivorship, you weave a story of versatility, trust, and strengthening. You are not characterized by malignant growth; you are characterized by your boldness, strength, and assurance to flourish past difficulty. Every day turns into a material — a material for flexibility, satisfaction, and reason.

Your process is a demonstration of the human soul's ability to rise, develop, and embrace life's intricacies with effortlessness and flexibility. As a cellular breakdown in the lungs survivor, you typify flexibility, trust, and the force of survivorship — a guide of motivation for others on their malignant growth venture.

Chapter 13

Advocacy and Patient Resources

Promotion for Cellular breakdown in the lungs Patients: A Voice for Mindfulness and Empowerment

Promotion is an integral asset for driving change, bringing issues to light, and engaging people and networks. As a cellular breakdown in the lungs patient or guardian, backing turns into a foundation of your journey — a stage to enhance your voice, advocate for further developed care and backing, and motivate positive change in the cellular breakdown in the lungs local area.

1. Figuring Out Advocacy

Backing is the most common way of shouting out, bringing issues to light, and making a move to resolve issues, advance change, and advance the interests of patients, guardians, and networks. It includes:

- **Raising Awareness: Teaching general society, policymakers, medical services experts, and the media about cellular breakdown in the lungs risk factors, avoidance procedures, screening rules, therapy choices, survivorship issues, and supportive resources.

- **Advancing Education: Enabling patients, guardians, and medical services experts with information, assets, and devices to settle on informed choices, access quality consideration, and explore the medical services framework successfully.

- **Driving Change: Pushing for strategy changes, research subsidizing, medical care access, fair consideration, patient-focused drives, and strong administrations that further develop results and personal satisfaction for cellular breakdown in the lungs patients.

2. The Job Of Advocates

Advocates assume a critical part in the cellular breakdown in the lungs local area, filling in as:

- **Voice of the Community: Backers enhance the voices of patients, parental figures, and medical care experts, sharing individual stories, encounters, difficulties, and necessities to drive change and bring issues to light.

- **Specialists of Change: Backers advocate for strategy changes, research financing, medical services access, survivorship support, and impartial consideration, collaborating with policymakers, administrators, medical care establishments, promotion associations, and local area partners.

- **Instructors and Resources: Promoters give training, assets, backing, and direction to patients, guardians, medical services experts, and people in general, enabling people with information, apparatuses, and procedures to explore the cellular breakdown in the lungs venture actually.

3. Promotion Strategies

Compelling promotion includes a scope of techniques and approaches, including:

- **Strategy Advocacy: Drawing in with policymakers, lawmakers, government offices, and promotion associations to advocate for approaches, regulation, subsidizing, and drives that focus on cellular breakdown in the lungs research, avoidance, early identification, treatment access, survivorship care, and steady administrations.

- **Local area Engagement: Building alliances, associations, and organizations inside the cellular breakdown in the lungs local area, teaming up with promotion associations, malignant growth habitats, medical care suppliers, support gatherings, and local area partners to arrange endeavors, share resources, and enhance influence.

- **Media and Mindfulness Campaigns: Utilizing media stages, online entertainment, advertising, mindfulness missions, occasions, and effort endeavors to bring issues to light, share data, destigmatize cellular breakdown in the lungs, advance early discovery, and feature patient stories and support drives.

- **Schooling and Empowerment: Giving instruction, assets, backing, and promotion preparing to patients, guardians, advocates, medical services experts, and the general population, enabling people with information, abilities, and apparatuses to advocate actually, explore the medical care framework, and access quality consideration.

Patient Assets and Backing Services

Notwithstanding promotion endeavors, cellular breakdown in the lungs patients approach a large number of assets and backing administrations intended to meet their novel requirements, improve their personal satisfaction, and give comprehensive consideration and backing. These assets include:

1. Disease Focuses and Treatment Facilities

- **Exhaustive Care: Malignant growth communities and therapy offices offer far reaching care, multidisciplinary groups, customized therapy plans, clinical preliminaries, steady administrations, and survivorship programs for cellular breakdown in the lungs patients.

- **Mastery and Specialization: Specific oncologists, pulmonologists, specialists, radiologists, attendants, social laborers, nutritionists, advisors, and care staff give skill, direction, and merciful consideration custom fitted to cellular breakdown in the lungs patients' necessities.

**2. Strong Consideration Services

- **Palliative Care: Palliative consideration groups center around alleviating side effects, overseeing aftereffects, working on personal satisfaction, tending to all encompassing requirements, and supporting patients and families all through the disease venture.

- **Psychosocial Support: Analysts, advocates, social specialists, and care groups offer daily encouragement, directing, survival methods, stress management, and resources to address mental, social, and otherworldly worries.

**3. Patient Schooling and Information

- **Instructive Resources: Malignant growth places, backing associations, and medical services suppliers offer instructive materials, online resources, online courses, studios, and educational meetings on cellular breakdown in the lungs, therapies, clinical preliminaries, survivorship, and strong consideration.

- **Clinical Preliminaries Information: Patients can get update about clinical preliminaries, research studies, exploratory therapies, and qualification models through malignant growth communities, clinical preliminary matching administrations, promotion associations, and online data sets.

**4. Monetary Help and Protection Support

- **Monetary Counseling: Monetary advisors, social specialists, and patient pilots give direction, resources, and help with exploring medical services costs, protection inclusion, monetary help programs, copayments, deductibles, and prescription expenses.

- **Patient Help Programs: Drug organizations, not-for-profit associations, government organizations, and backing bunches offer patient help programs, copay help, medicine limits, and monetary guide for qualified patients.

**5. Survivorship and Health Programs

- **Survivorship Care: Survivorship projects, facilities, and administrations center around long haul follow-up care, observing, survivorship care plans, late pain impact, health methodologies, daily encouragement, and resources for disease survivors.

- **Health and Integrative Therapies: Integrative medication programs, health focuses, and correlative treatments, for example, needle therapy, rub treatment, yoga, contemplation, nourishment advising, and practice programs advance comprehensive wellbeing, side effect of the pain and personal satisfaction.

**6. Local area Resources And Backing Groups

- **Support Groups: Cellular breakdown in the lungs support gatherings, online networks, peer support projects, and parental figure support administrations offer everyday reassurance, peer associations, data sharing, methods for dealing with stress, and assets for patients, survivors, guardians, and families.

- **Local area Resources: Nearby associations, philanthropies, backing gatherings, malignant growth social orders, and public venues give outreach, training, promotion, monetary guide, transportation administrations, lodging help, dinner conveyance, and functional help for disease patients and families.

Conclusion: Supporters, Informed Patients

As a cellular breakdown in the lungs patient, guardian, or backer, you approach an abundance of resources, support administrations, and promotion open doors that enable you to explore the cellular breakdown in the lungs venture really, access quality consideration, advocate for change, and further develop results for you and others.

By utilizing promotion techniques, drawing in with patient resources, and working together with medical care experts, backing associations, and local area partners, you become an enabled advocate, informed patient, and impetus for positive change in the cellular breakdown in the lungs local area.

Together, through backing, education, backing, and strengthening, we can bring issues to light, drive progress, and change the scene of cellular breakdown in the lungs care and backing, guaranteeing that each patient gets the empathy, care, and resources they merit.

Acknowledgement

I wish to thank Almighty God for the inspiration to undertake this project and contribute to the society positively.

About the Author

Leo Chambers is a creative writer and Digital Content Creator.